# I THOUGHT I WAS THE KING OF SCOTLAND

## *Jimmy Gilmour*

**chipmunkapublishing**
the mental health publisher
empowering people with bi-polar manic
depression

Jimmy Gilmour

Published by
Chipmunkapublishing
PO Box 6872
Brentwood
Essex CM13 1ZT
United Kingdom

**http://www.chipmunkapublishing.com**

Edited by Debra Shulkes

I

Chipmunkapublishing gratefully acknowledges the support of Arts Council England.

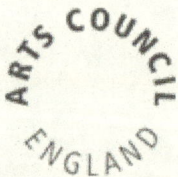

## ACKNOWLEDGEMENTS

Thank you to my wife Janet
And her family and good friends
And my Daughter Jemma


CARE SPECIALISTS

The Staff at the
Carlton Hayes Hospital
Bradgate unit Glenfied Hospital
And CPN's who looked after me
And also The Leicester General Hospital

# Jimmy Gilmour

# I THOUGHT I WAS THE KING OF SCOTLAND

Why did I write this book?
James the King of Scotland.

This is who I thought I would be. I knew I would be able to write a small book after my second breakdown, but I am not very good at wording things, but I have tried my best. These false beliefs went on until my fifth breakdown. I am not a nutter and I am not mad I just wanted to share my experiences with people that have had similar experiences in life.

By writing this book I thought I would find out where the King of Scotland really came from and put an end to all these false beliefs. I have been through a long and painful journey having Bi-Polar Disorder, then being wrongly diagnosed more than once then being back to Bi-Polar Disorder again.

I have had five nervous breakdowns since 1995 and lost my family and friends, it took me two years after my breakdown to regain my confidence again and get my life back together. After drinking heavily in the past and suicide attempts and over spending money. I never thought I would get married again and have a new family and friends.

I hope the experiences that I have shared with you will be helpful to fellow service users, professionals and people out in the community. To help with the stigma of mental health.

I want people to understand more about mental health problems.

# Jimmy Gilmour

# I THOUGHT I WAS THE KING OF SCOTLAND

## CHAPTER ONE

Born in Ayr Scotland

I was born on the 21$^{st}$ of October 1961, in a place called Kilwinning in Scotland. My mother and father met each other five years before my birth. My father was a bus driver and my mother was the conductor and that's how they came to meet each other. Within the five years before my birth my mother and father moved houses approximately a hundred times around Glasgow and Ayrshire.

In 1963 me my mother and father moved to England to a place called Thringstone on a Scottish estate, in a two bed roomed flat. Along with us a lot of other Scottish and Gordie families moved to that area to work down the pits. That's where my father took on his first job in England as a mineworker in Whitwick pit. He worked there for twelve months and didn't like the conditions underground and he left and started to work as a lorry driver. Soon after that his cab caught on fire and inside was his jacket with his weeks wages, which at the time was the least of his worries as the lorry went up in flames. With him being worried about money trying to keep a roof over his wife and sons head, it caused him to become stressed he had a nervous breakdown. He ended up in a psychiatric hospital, Carlton Hayes. He was sectioned for twenty-eight days. The doctors diagnosed him with Post Traumatic Stress

Syndrome. Not long after he came out of hospital with the stigma that is attached to mental health he wanted to go back to Scotland, and told his wife that he wanted to take his son James. This caused them both to have a big argument about taking me to Scotland. It was around Christmas time and all a can remember is crying in the kitchen. The argument passed and my father stayed with us in Thringstone.

In 1965 my mother fell pregnant and in October 1966 she gave birth to my sister. With us living in a small flat we then had to move to a three bed roomed house still living on the Scottish estate. Everything seemed to be fine until 1971 my father just left without any goodbyes, at the time my mother was at work and me my sister were still sleeping, this all seems all a blur to me. We all assumed that he had gone back to Scotland. My mother later divorced him. In 1973 she met another man who had five daughters and two sons where we went to live with them in a four bed roomed house still on the Scottish estate. The majority of his children moved back to Scotland to go and live with their mother. The rest made their own lives in England. Which then left four of us me, my sister, my mother and her partner then had to move again because the house was to big for us, also the council wanted us to move back to a three bed roomed house because it was needed by larger families. We still found ourselves living on the Scottish estate swapping our house with a larger family.

In 1977 I left school with no qualifications and that's when a started to work down Snibston colliery. Within a month of me working my father visited us one morning and wanted to know if he was divorced to my mother. She was at work at the time at Loughborough hospital nursing. He spoke to my mother via telephone and an argument erupted where he then found out that he was divorced, she told him to stay away. I realised who he was but he never spoke one word to me he just left with no goodbyes. In 1978 I pass my driving test, my grandma died at a early age I didn't really know her that much with me being young, but I knew my granddad and later on he passed away and a took my mother and her partner to the funeral in Commack Scotland.

I tuned eighteen a year after in 1979 my local pub was the Rose and Crown in Thringstone. My hobbies were water skiing, playing pool and playing football with the lads. I enjoyed life in Thringstone and had a group of good and trustworthy friends.

In 1984 I left home and brought a house in Thringstone where I lived with my girlfriend a year later in October 1985 we got married in Ibstock and had a full Scottish wedding wearing a kilt. Then on the 24th of March 1988 my wife gave birth to my daughter, Jemma. Which was the happiest day of my life. The house that I had earlier brought was £17,000 and in 1989 it went up to £60,000. My wife wanted to move to Ibstock to be near her mother because I was working at Asfordby mine at the time in a three shift pattern, six days a week with a week off. Where I left all my childhood friends behind.

# Jimmy Gilmour

## British Coal

I left school at sixteen and went to work at Snibston Colliery where I had to do a twelve-week training course at Burch Copies – this was in March 1977. I had to learn how to do the safety underground and work the tools. When I finished my twelve weeks course I started Snibston Colliery in June, my first job underground was at the pit bottom taking the supplies in and out the pit bottom. My first wage packet was £**26.00** pound a week, my shift pattern was 7 hours and 15 minutes, days and afternoons starting at 7 in the morning until quarter past 2 in the afternoon and 2 till 10 on the afternoon shift.

After finishing working at the pit bottom I went on supplies until I was 18 and then had to do a 3 months training course on the coalface. Working down the pit was a tough life with conditions underground being difficult, I enjoyed working underground with other miners. Then I started working on the coalface doing chocking and snaking and in the stables on a yard seem.

Snibston colliery was in a town called Coalville it was due to close so I transferred to Ellistown colliery in 1983, there give the men **£1,500** to transfer which was paid at **£500.00** every 6 months.

I was working on the coalface and a 1 years later I worked in the headings where I drove a machine called a 'JCM', which stands for Joy Contenting Mining.

# I THOUGHT I WAS THE KING OF SCOTLAND

In 1984 the miners went on strike I was in the num a lot of miners from Yorkshire came to Leicestershire to picket the mines all over Leicestershire. But some miners continued to work and were branded as scabs by there colleagues when they crossed the picket line, a lot of police from London came to Ellistown colliery for the safety of the miners who crossed the picket line.

A lot of miners travelled to London Hyde Park to listen a great speaker who was also our NUM leader, which was a good day out we walked through London with banners protesting that the government wanted to close the pits all over the country and the strike ending a year later which got a lot of miners in debt and lost their homes.

I still continued to work at Ellistown colliery until 1989 when it was due to close I had an option of two pits Door mill or Asfordby mine - I chose Asfordby mine.

Asfordby Mine

In 1989, I started three shift patterns - days afternoon and nights and then a week off to work at Asfordby mine the contractors sunk the shafts there were a lot of Irish men there as contractors, my tally number was 11 for a start there was not many of us there, our first job was at the pit tops in the work shops building up JCM to see if they worked properly. Then we dismantle them then they had to go to the pit bottom, our second job was to build some platforms underground the wages were **£400.00** a week, which was good for a start. Then after we built the platforms then we started to build the JCM underground, the contractors were finished doing their work. We started doing headings with steel and roof bolts and the JCM would load the coal into a shuttle car which hold 11 tonnes of coal and the road ways were 15ft wide and 8ft high, then after 12 months we came off steel and just went on roof bolts we used wombats resin and roof bolts and wire meshing in 1992 we started to earn a lot of money top line was **£1,000** a week and we worked very hard for it and I was glad for the week off, I had a lot of good friends there, **400** miners from the Leicestershire pits and Derbyshire.

Being a miner was a big part of my life and I thought I had a job for life, it cost British Coal a lot of money to build Asfordby mine in Melton Mowbray. A lot of miners who worked there moved location to be near work, I lived in Ibstock at the time and had to travel 24 miles one way. It came a shock to me when I heard they where going to close down the mine, then I had to make the biggest decision of my life - to go to Doormill or take redundancies - and I choose to take the redundancy payment On December 4th 1993.

CHAPTER TWO

Living in Ibstock.

In 1990 I took my family to Tenerife Porterico, over there I met friends from Ibstock and stayed in the same hotel as them. I then started to make new friends in Ibstock and my local pub then was the Ram. In 1992 I was still working at Asfordby mine on a afternoon shift and went for a drink with a couple of friends to a night club in Griffydam. I had three bottles of Budweiser, my friend took me home to Ibstock I was hungry that night and couldn't be bothered to make anything to eat. So I took the risk and jumped into my car and drove to Coalville for an Indian and I passed a police car. The police car turned on its blue lights and started to follow me, I lost them for a start but them they traced me and caught me. I had to follow the normal police procedure and take a breathalyser test, this really shook me up as my diving license were valuable to me for many of reasons. I failed the breathalyser test and they took my to Loughborough police station because Coalville police station was under going decoration. Where there a blew into a machine that told the police officers how much I was over. Over the limited so had to appear in court a month later. I lost my driving license in 1993 for twelve months. This is where my life started to go down hill.

On December the 4th 1993 I took redundancy from British coal. I waited until Christmas and New Year passed by and in January I took my forklift driving licence and passed. I then applied for twelve jobs over a period of eleven months; I had three interviews out the twelve but never got any of the jobs. My head started to take a lot of battering I started to panic because I was out of work and I started to drink heavily. In that year I had two holidays abroad, one on a stag week to Magaluff with thirty-two lads from ibstock. I knew by that time that there was something wrong with me, I was drinking a lot and become high and it was due to over spending. The deal was if I went on holiday I would have to take my wife and daughter to Spain when I came back, which we did two months after my return home. In Spain I came to my senses and realised that my marriage was all over. When we returned back to Ibstock I lived with my wife and daughter until I found a job, I then started to work at Ibstock brickyard. I left it until

Christmas was over to make sure that I had some good memories of our last Christmas together. I had planned in my mind that I was going to leave home New Years eve, but I started to loose sleep and wasn't strong enough.

On January the 5th 1995 I went to my GP's and asked for sleeping tablets and the doctor was to concerned about my blood. The next day the doctor came to visit me and asked me if there was any where I could go to get away from all the trouble, but I had no where to go because I lost contact with my mum in 1990. My wives brother took me to my mothers and she saw the state I was in and took me in.

Friday 6th January I arrived at my mother's house at around 7pm, I told her my marriage was breaking down and things between us hadn't been good since 1993. My mum asked me why I had not visited her in four years, and went on to explain how I thought she felt. I thought that she wasn't interested about my daughter and also knew if I visited her on a regular basis she would pick up that there were something wrong with my marriage. I know how strict my mum can be and knew she would say you have made your bed now lie in it and that I should never have left Thringstone. She saw that I was in a state and was heading for a breakdown, with her being a nurse. I started to get all agitated due to lack of sleep, I then went on to telling her that I had started to drink heavily and had took redundancy from British coal. She then went onto asking me how much money I had left. I told her that I had three thousand pounds to my name. Mum started to fire questions at me about my marriage and I explained that we had been sleeping in separate bedrooms and that we had even tried marriage guidance for the sake of our daughter, and but it didn't work.

I was hurting inside and I felt really bad, as I had not seen both my mother and sister now for four years. I didn't sleep very well that night, as it felt strange sleeping back at mums house after all those years. Saturday morning around 11am my wife pulled up outside, she came in and asked my mum if she could borrow the telephone. She handed over five pounds to my mum for letting her use the phone, she had phoned the doctors up, the doctors advised her to take me back home. Before leaving for home my mum and wife started to argue so my step dad told me to go upstairs out the way. That's when mum must have realised that I needed professional help. I felt very vulnerable; I walked into the car with my wife to go home. I noticed that my diary was in the door panel, and couldn't understand why it was there. Not one word was spoken between both of us on the journey home. We went inside to the house when we arrived my wife had my diary in her hand; she then went outside and gave the diary to her mother who then drove off. Something triggered in my brain there were a lot of my friends phone numbers in that diary. So I rang the police and told them that someone had stole my diary. When the police arrived at my house they could sense that there was something wrong with me and that I was not very well at all. So they got two doctors and a social worker to come and see me. There were two policemen one in my kitchen and one outside, they told me that I had to stay where I was until the doctors arrived. The time seemed to be dragging and felt like that I was waiting for ages. When they turned up they were two psychiatrists with black bags. The social worker told me to speak to the psychiatrist; I really can't remember what I said to them because by that time my head had completely gone.

# I THOUGHT I WAS THE KING OF SCOTLAND

Things all seemed so strange to me, I was very scared because there were a lot of people in my room. The doctors told me that I had to wait for a ambulance to come. When it arrived I just walked out of the house and got into it out of my own free will. Just before the doors shut my wife's brother said are you going to say anything? And all I replied was money. After we had been travelling a few miles it then came to my senses to ask them where I was going, and they turned round and said to me we are taking you to Carlton-Hayes Hospital.

# CHAPTER THREE

Carlton-Hayes Hospital.

I arrived at Carlton-Hayes hospital, the ambulance driver took me onto the ward and they informed me that I was staying on ward KC5. I first seen a nurse she asked me a variety of questions like 'Do you know where you are?' and 'Do you know what's wrong with you?' she told me that she had got a bed ready for me to stay in. I told her that my marriage had broken down, I had been drinking heavily and had became very agitated and had problems sleeping. She then took me up stairs to my dormitory; there were around twenty beds in there. The nurse had to follow their normal procedure and check my bags and wrote down what I had brought in with me in case I had any things that I shouldn't have. Everything seemed a blur to me as I was not thinking straight and everything happened so fast. Then I went back downstairs on the ward, there I met another nurse that started to ask me questions and they seemed to be the same as what the other nurse told me. They said that they would give me some sleeping pills, which would help me sleep, they were called Temazepan. And informed me that I would not be able to see a doctor until Monday afternoon. The only thing that I could remember after that was they gave me some drinking chocolate and then I went to bed.

# I THOUGHT I WAS THE KING OF SCOTLAND

I slept a little that night. I got up in the morning to have a shave and I felt that somebody's presents had been there before. It was my Dad. But I didn't know if this was because I was paranoid and hallucinating. This time I thought that I was loosing my mind. I didn't want to tell any of the nurses about it, and then I went and had breakfast. After breakfast I went to ring my mother, she said that she would come and visit me in the afternoon and all the family would be there. The nurses were talking to me but they wouldn't tell me where I was, so after dinner when my mother and family came we all sat around that table and I asked mum where I was, and she said you're in a mental hospital. I Replied 'What the Looney bin?' by then I knew where I was. We all gathered hands and some of us cried, mum said that she would come back tomorrow so that she could see the doctor.

I asked the nurse if I could have some fresh air and they said that you would not be able to go out until you have seen the doctor tomorrow. I couldn't bring myself to talk to the other patients, so I just watched television. After a while I rang my best friend up and told him where I was and he said 'I thought it was you!' we saw the ambulance outside your house. I asked him to visit but not to come until I had been there for a week. That night I took my medication as prescribed and went to bed. I was still having racing thoughts due to paranoia. I couldn't wait until I have seen the consultant the next day and I thought to myself 'Well Jim your in a mental hospital, my brain has been through a lot! You need a rest!' I managed to get four hours sleep. The next morning I had my breakfast, and that I could think about was getting some fresh air.

Time seemed to drag on that day but after dinner I saw the consultant. He said to me what's brought you here? I replied 'Marriage breakdown, spending a lot of money, drinking heavily at weekends and taking redundancy from British coal'. There were too many people in with the doctor. I felt out of control and I felt that my life was in their hands. The doctor prescribed me some medication, Carbamazepine and to carry on taking the sleeping pills. The doctor asked if it was all right to speak to my mother, and I said yes. After mum had spoken to the doctor she came to talk to me for a while before she left. The doctor said I was allowed off the ward twice a day fifteen minutes each time with supervision. The hospital had four acres of land and lovely gardens, when I was outside I realised it was an old asylum. I had a next meeting with the consultant on the Wednesday and that's when he asked me if he could see my wife, to make sure that what I have told the doctor and nurses were true. My wife came into the hospital and I made her a drink, then she had to go and see the doctor. Once she had left the doctor, it was my turn to go back in. My wife had told the doctor to tell me that my marriage was over and that I was never to go back to the house again and I needed to find some place else to live.

After I saw the doctor, I remember walking to the hospital shops, they were long straight corridors that went on for about a quarter of a mile. Then somebody told me where the kitchen was, it took half an hour for the trolley to reach KC5, and when it did the food wasn't very nice at all. It was nice to be able to walk around the hospital on my own, but I still wasn't allowed to walk the hospital grounds unsupervised.

The 14th January I had been in hospital for a week now and started to feel better in myself and more relaxed. I was looking forwards to my friends coming to visit me. After I had eaten my dinner sixteen lads from Ibstock came in to see me, it made me feel happy and lifted me for a while. Having quieted a few visitors the nurse said that they could take me for a drink down the pub. There were ten more of my friends waiting for me, as they had been playing football in Ender by. One of my friends said to me 'sorry I didn't visit you in hospital Jimmy I didn't think I would be able to handle it'. My best friend told me that my job was safe. After we had had a couple of drinks they took me back to the hospital. The next day I saw the doctor again and he increased my medication from 400mg to 600mg of Carbamazepine daily. I was still taking Temazepan as well, the doctor his self could she that I was a lot better than when I first arrived in hospital. Seeing that I was a lot better he told me that I was allowed to walk the gardens on my own. This made me feel more relaxed. Then the next step was for me to ask the doctor if I could leave the hospital grounds on my own. I started to talk to the other patients and played pool with them, and asked them what had brought them in here. I was feeling that I had more control over my life now, I was sleeping better and not so agitated. The nurses could see that I was improving a lot so they let me take a trip to the nearest town centre on my own. I found a fitness centre near by so the next day I was let off the ward for three hours and went swimming.

Every morning of me being at the hospital I used to wake up have my breakfast and walk around the hospital grounds as I loved the fresh air, it made me think and feel better. Then it would be lunchtime and after lunch I would go down into the town with other patients. Later on in the day I would go for a drink and be back for ten pm, for medication and bed. The next time I saw the doctor it was Wednesday he asked me how I was. I told him that I was well, so he said on Friday I could have leave for the weekend and return back to the hospital on the Sunday afternoon, but that I would have to take some extra medication as I would be out in the community.

When I went on leave on Friday afternoon, I went to stay with my mother, she gave me the extra tablet of which the doctor had prescribed for me, I can't remember what it was called, but it was blue. After I had taken my first tablet around ten minuets after I wanted another so I ended up taking four or five more than I should have done. They made me feel all agitated and I didn't sleep very well that night. Then on the Saturday morning I couldn't handle things, so my step dad took me back to the hospital. I didn't like it one bit that I was back on the ward. So I had to see the doctor the next day. There were a lot of people in there; the doctor asked me what was up with me. And I told him that I feel as though I am back to square one again. He told me that he would give me something to make me feel better a depot injection so he changed my medication from Carbamazepine tablets to a depixol injection. So the nurses gave me the injection and asked me if I felt better, and I replied yes. I knew nothing about the 1983 mental health act, and I didn't realise at the time that I was on a section two, which is a twenty-eight day section where your not able to leave the hospital without your section finished. The doctor told me that I would have to have the injection every two weeks and it would keep me out of the hospital, and everything else that is wrong with you we can fix that too. The depot seemed to be working I just felt a bit agitated and muscle stiffness, I didn't realise that it were the side effects from the depot, and so they gave me some Procyclidine.

When I saw the doctor again he could see that I was much better and my section of twenty-eight days had finished. So he said that I was free to leave. I went to stay with my mother and stepfather so they helped me get a flat in Coalville. But I felt at the time that I wasn't ready for it, and there had been many changes already in my life, and I felt I wasn't ready to handle it on my own. It cost me £1,000 to start my own flat up and I started back to work at Ibstock brickyard. Making concrete window cells and plenty more things. I found it harder work than when I was working down the pit. The first Friday I was out of hospital I went for a drink with my friends. But living in Coalville I felt isolated and my sleep started to go down hill, and I wasn't taking my Procyclidine properly. Two weeks later I had to go to my GP's for my injection. Then I went o to see my mother and she told me that she had my divorce papers for me. So then I had to get a solicitor for my divorce and sort out some maintenance for my daughter. I carried on working but I didn't feel myself, I was sweating a lot at work, not sleeping very well, couldn't concentrate on the television and my diet wasn't very good at all. By now it was March 1995 on the Saturday I told my wife that my daughter could sleep over at the flat the next week, as I had got her room ready for her and that I would pick her up at around six at night.

By Wednesday, at work in the morning I went to have my breakfast but I could not eat it as I felt really sick, the lads told me to go and lie down in the first aid room for a bit. But my work mates realised that I was unwell, so they took me to see my mum, but she wasn't in she was out shopping. So they took me back to my flat and my friends told me to make sure that I was to go back to my mother's house to see her when she was back. When I went back to mums she asked me what was wrong with me and told me I was staring and she didn't like it. At this time I was feeling very suicidal but couldn't bring myself to telling my mum. I didn't want to go back to the hospital so I got my car and went back to the flat. When I got home I shut myself out from the outside world, I did not answer the telephone, and I thought why am I suicidal? This was going through my brain over and over again for three whole days and three nights. All I could think about was if there was a shotgun in this flat? And if there were I wouldn't be here now. And I kept thinking to myself I am picking my daughter up on Saturday at 6pm. What would my friends and family think if I committed suicide? This was going over and over like a record in my mind, but only a fellow sufferer or a specialist would understand the mental pain that I was experiencing. I found a knife and started to cut at my right arm to see if all the pain out of my head would disappear. So I went into the kitchen got a pint glass and smashed it in the sink I took pieces of glass with me into the living room and sat on a little step. With my right hand as it was much stringer than my left I cut my skin open it was midday on the Saturday that I was meant to be seeing my daughter. I was cutting away and the blood was all up the walls. I started to cut through my tendons then I started to feel better, my brain was clean, by then I knew I had lost my sanity.

It was getting on for 6pm, my jeans were soaked with blood, I went into the kitchen and got a tea towel, wrapped it around my wrist. There was blood all over the kitchen floor. I knew that I had to ring for an ambulance, so I did and on the phone I told them that I tried to commit suicide. The police arrived first they looked around the flat to see if anyone else was there. I told them that I had done this to myself, the ambulance arrived they strapped my wrist up and they took me to the hospital. The nurse at the hospital said has a woman done this to you? I did not answer. The nurse came to see me they thought they could just stitch me up but then they realised I needed an operation because I had damaged my tendons in my wrist. I had been in the hospital for three days before my mother and sister came to see me I just told my mum that I was sorry for what I had done. After the surgeons had operated on me and put it in plaster they told me that I would only have ninety-five per cent of feeling in my left hand. I had so much burning pain in my heart that my working days were over. What would people think with the stigma of mental health? Then my social worker and CPN came to visit me. They told me that the psychiatrist wanted to see me at the hawthorn centre. The consultant said that I had to go back into the hospital again  love hurts.

CHAPTER FOUR

Carlton Hayes Hospital, The second time.

There I was at the Hawthorn centre, I felt all Alone and a sorry, sorry sight for a man.
Then the CPN and the social worker came to me and they took me in the car back to Carlton Hayes Hospital. All I could feel at the time was a lot of anxiety, and was getting very stiff because of the lack of Procyclidine which I hadn't had for about three to four days. I was anxious and worried about what people might think about me trying to commit suicide. We arrived at KC5 ward they sat me outside the office, the nurse held my hand. The doctors were deciding what to do with me, whether to give me the injection or ECT treatment and this was going on for a long time. I thought I was going to die.... They decide to give me the injection, Depixol again. Then I went up to the dormitory and the doctor came to see me and ask me some questions. He asked me who the Prime minister was? And I told him who it was! He asked me to count backwards from twenty, which I struggled on. Then he asked me to say the alphabet backwards, and replied you've got no chance. I was feeling very low at this time; the trembling gradually went away because I had had the injection. I went to lie on my bed and I couldn't wait until it was night time because I just wanted to die in my sleep. Then the nurse said to me Jimmy your mum is here. I walked down to the bottom of

the stairs and my mum gave me a bic razor blade and told me to keep the shaver going, and I knew what she meant that I had to hold onto my dignity. I took it upstairs then after that I went back down stairs to talk to my mother, but my speech was very slurred and I couldn't speak because I was that low, so mum left and I went back to my bed.

All I could think about was that I couldn't wait until night time until I get my sleeping pills, because I wanted to die in my sleep. I stayed in bed and the nurse came up at night time to give me my medication and told me that I was to see the doctor tomorrow afternoon. I didn't even get one-hour sleep because I was very agitated and all worked up seeing the doctor. Morning came and I had a shave and managed to get myself in the bath, it was hard with having my wrist in plaster. It was hard to get dressed on my own I knew I had to keep doing this if I got any chance of getting out of hospital this time. I went downstairs for some breakfast but couldn't eat any so I went back to bed, and I was still waiting for night time to come. By this time the nurse came up to me and told me that I had to go and see the doctor. There were around twenty people in with the doctor; I felt all-alone the doctor said to me you have got friends! You have got family! You've got a job why try and take you life? And I couldn't answer him. He upped my sleeping pills, Temazepan to forty mg and he also gave me Chlorpromazine twenty mg and then I left the room. I went straight back to bed I felt self-worthless. How was I going to get through this one?

# I THOUGHT I WAS THE KING OF SCOTLAND

My mum and sister came to visit me again it was the second week in March 1995, it was a nice day and the sun was out. Mum said to me if you want this to be your life this will always be your life. I knew she was trying to help me, then the ward manager came to us and he said the doctor said you need an antidepressant to lift your mood. And I said what's that? Seroxat he said it's the only thing that will get you out of this hospital, and I said have I got to come off the depo injection? No he said you have to keep taking that as well so I said ok! Only if it would get me out of here. My mum left and I rang up my wife to see if she would bring in my daughter so that I could see her she told me that she would bring her on Sunday.

The wife didn't like the coffee so she brought her own flask, I can remember my daughter, playing pool, and I don't think she knew really what was going off. The wife upset me because all she wanted was maintenance off me for my daughter so the nurse asked her to leave. I didn't realised that I was being watched constantly, I went to bed that night and I managed to get four hours sleep I was no longer thinking about dying in my sleep.

The first two weeks I was there I didn't think about getting any fresh air at all. Then the third Wednesday there I had to see the doctor again. I asked him if could just go around the ground for half an hour. He also asked me how my sleep was? I told him that I was sleeping for four hours, which I thought the medication they were giving me would knock an elephant out. I didn't ring any friends up until the third week, and I told my best friend that he could come and see me on the

Friday night. I told him what I had done and he said to me that I need professional help and that he would visit me on the Friday night. I started talking to some of the patients in there; some were still in there from last time. The nurse allowed me to go into the town centre when my friends came to visit me on the Friday night with them, but they didn't say much because they couldn't understand the mental pain I was going through. It felt as if I only had two friends left in Ibstock. They made sure that I was back to the hospital by ten o'clock. Which then I had my medication and went to bed.

 The next day I started to mix more with the patients and started to play pool. They let me go outside for some fresh air, I looked at the front entrance of the Asylum and I thought to myself that I was never going to get out of here because I felt that there were no change in myself. By now I had been in hospital for four weeks coming up to the end of my section two. I went to see the doctor again. To ask about having the plaster taken off of my wrist, Which I had to go to the hospital for them to take it off and for them to check it out. When I had had that done and was back in Carlton Hayes I rang my mum up to ask her if she could get me out of hospital. She said to me that I had to wait for my twenty-eight days were up so that I could get my papers. I didn't realise at the time that I only had two days left until the end of my section. A nurse tapped me on the shoulder and told me that I was free to leave but I had to see the doctor first. The doctor told me that I had to carry on taking the depot injection and I would stay out in the community. I said yes doctor. So I

# I THOUGHT I WAS THE KING OF SCOTLAND

left the hospital and went to stay with my mother
and step dad, as why I was in hospital my mother
had let my flat go, because I wasn't able to cope
on my own.

## CHAPTER FIVE

Back at Mums

First week in April 1995 at mum's house, it felt all so strange at first going back to live there after being in hospital for four weeks. Mum told me that I had lost my three hundred pound deposit that I had put down on the flat. I told her not to worry about it. My arm was still in a sling and I had to go hospital the week after to have some physiotherapy, I went and lay in bed just thinking, just wishing that I was someone else. Racing thoughts going threw my mind just like a record playing over and over again and I just wanted them to stop. I was paranoid about all the medication that I was taking. Why does this have to happen to me? What had I done to deserve this? Mum shouted me down for dinner I couldn't eat a lot, and I couldn't understand why they let me out the hospital? I watched some television but I couldn't concentrate I didn't even know what channel I was watching. I took my medication and went to bed I didn't get much sleep as per usual as I was agitated these were the side affects from the medication and lack of sleep.

I was suffering from anxiety and deep depression. Saturday morning came I ate a little breakfast then went back to bed. Mum woke me up and bathed me. I just knew I was a complete vegetable at this time. I sat down on the settee and spoke to mum for a while as my step dad had gone out. Mum told me that she had to clean the blood up in the flat; I replied that couldn't have been easy for you. And she said you shouldn't be alive and that I could rock the barrels. I didn't understand at the time what she was going on about, but I don't know what I would have done without her. I knew that she would have to look after me for a long while, as I needed a lot of TLC. My pattern was like this for a full week.

The Saturday after I rang my best friend up from Ibstock and I told him that I was out of hospital. He said that he would come and pick you up in half an hour. He took me straight to The Ram a pub in Ibstock I felt so embarrassed and guilty. Some of my friends where in the pub, they came over and spoke to me and shook my hand and said that it was a very brave thing that I had tried to do. I knew that my best friend had put me straight in at the deep end. Having to face all my friends, he said that I knew you would be able to do this Jimmy. I had a couple of pints then he took me back to mum's house. On the Monday morning I had to go for physiotherapy looking down at what I had done to my wrist made me feel more anxious. They strapped it back up and told me that I would have to get a ball and do plenty of exercises with it else I wouldn't be able to pick a shopping bag up with it. I went back to mums still depressed I wasn't bothered about getting any fresh air; the circulation in my legs wasn't very good. They started to get stiffer and stiffer.

Me and mum talked a lot she went upstairs and came back down with a letter, it was form my dad he had wrote it several years ago when I was fifteen and my sister was ten. I was thirty-three now and she had never told us about the letter, he had wrote asking to see us. He was living in London. He wanted mum to put my sister and me on a train at Loughborough and he would meet us off the train in London Station, and that he had some money to give us both. When she told me I felt that I had missed out a lot in life with visits. Then mum told me that when I was three years old they had both had a big row because my father didn't like living in England and wanted to go back to Scotland. He wanted to take me with him but she wouldn't let him. She also told me that I was just like my dad I didn't know what to think at the time with my head being in a mess. But I've got a good memory. I went to bed, not long after my mum shouted up and told me that dinner was done. I had been feeling depressed for two weeks now, the reason why I didn't want to go outside was because my wrist was still in bandages, and I didn't know what people in Thringstone would think with the stigma of mental health.

I was glad that I had to go back to Leicester Royal for the last time. They took my bandages off. I got back home and I was due to have my two-week depot injection at my GP'S in Ibstock. It was the first time that I had driven my car for a while. I was still taking my other medications, which were Depixo, Chlorpromazine, Procyclidine, Temazepan and Seroxat. Friday night third week in April 1995, I went to meet my friend in the pub in Ibstock. I only had a glass of coke.

At about ten o'clock I had suicidal thoughts and tendencies to connect the Hoover pipe to the exhaust. I knew I had to go back to mums as she had an upright Hoover under the stairs with extensions that I could use. I was fighting the suicidal thoughts and tendencies while I was driving I pulled up a quarter of a mile away from Thringstone near a farm called Sharply Rocks I got in and out the car several times my brain was in turmoil going over and over again the mental pain I was in, just like a tape playing. I got out of the car again this time I banged my firsts on the grass and said God where the Fucking Hell are you? We cannot let this happen again I looked up at the stars and banged on the bonnet of the car with my fists and I got back into the car and burst out crying and the suicidal thoughts went, and I dried my tears then drove my car back to mums and went straight to bed.

I knew I had to make a big decision about coming off one of my tablets this went on all night and I did not get any sleep, I decided to come off the Chlorpromazine because I was still needed the antidepressant if I had any chance of lifting my mood and getting out of this depression. I did not tell my mother I was coming off one of my tablets, I just pretended to swallow it and kept it up the roof of my mouth and then flushed it down the toilet.

In May I told my mum that I had come off the Chlorpomazine, she said you better not come off the injection or your antidepressant, if you do you will end up back in hospital and am not looking after you, I knew myself I had to keep on them as I was still suicidal. The suicidal thoughts would come and go.

I contacted my solicitor because my divorce was on hold, to sign some papers he told me it would only take four months then I would be divorced, and I can remember signing and feeling suicidal and staring and shaking and blurred vision, with mental pain I could not wait to get out the room, I drove back to mums house and went straight to bed. The next day I rang up the wife to see if I could have Jemma then I took her to Bosworth Park, it was a good way to keep my mind busy and also see my daughter as I felt she was keeping me going. In the school holidays I seen more of my daughter and the wife said what again but she never stopped me from seeing her.

I was still getting sick pay from Ibstock brick yard, I received one hundred and twenty pound a week I knew myself there was no way I could get back to work being on this injection because I had poor concentration and no confidence in myself to get back to work, but they could not sack me until the doctor had signed off the club.

In June I went to see my GP and asked him to sign me off the club so I could go back to work he told me I did not have to go back to work that I could stay on the club, but I wanted him to sign me off.

I went to see my boss at Ibstock brick yard he said I have been though a divorce and I cannot understand what its done to you I am sorry but I have got to sack you I was glad because I felt guilty taking the money because I had not worked there for very long. A couple of days later my sleep was not very good I made to visits to the shop and brought some Paracetamol, I knew I was going to miss working with my friends I could not see any future me being stuck at mums for the rest of my life and living on benefits.

I had 64 paracetamols laid out on my bed I swallowed three of them then I said to myself what ever going wrong in my life I was determined to fight this mental pain what I was going through and to stay alive, I put the paracetamols away and went for a long walk to clear my head to the Monastery which was three miles away from mums house, and to get the negative thoughts out my head. I walked back to mums house and I started to feel a bit better, the school holidays had finished.

I went to visit my friends in Ibstock we would go out every Friday for a drink and every Sunday for dinner.

Christmas came and I was still living with my mother and I was glad that I would not have to spend Christmas on my own, everybody looked happy except me I did not want to be taking depixol it made me depressed just being on it, I just felt like a zombie, after the new year I went to see my CPN who I had to see every two weeks at the Hawthorne Centre, I told her that I had over stayed my welcome at mums and that I wanted to come off the injection she said she would have to see the doctor first.

First week in March 1996 I started to go to the Travellers Rest night club I thought dancing would do me good as I enjoyed dancing. I met a woman and she asked me for a lift home she lived in Nuneaton thirty miles away, when I dropped her off she gave me her telephone number. The following Saturday I went to the Travellers rest with my friends, the woman who I had met the week before was there, she told me she'd not long been out a violent relationship and moved away to Nuneaton to get away from him. I told her I was going through a divorce, she asked me if I would give her a lift home she asked me if I was working and I just said yes. When we arrived at her house I asked her if I could stay for the week she said yes I got myself some toiletries from the shop, my medication was at mums house.

At the end of the week the phone went it was my CPN mum must have found the number in my bedroom and gave it to her she asked me if I was all right and if I would come back and see her at the Hawthorne centre.

I was not feeling too good because I had come off the seroxat all at once. I got back to mums house and I had to go to my GPs at Ibstock to get my injection. Mum told me while I was away she had changed my doctors to Whitwick so I went there to get my injection then I had to go to the Hawthorne centre to see my CPN I told that I had come off the Chlorpromazine and Seroxat. She said why have you done that because of all the side effects, and also I want to come off the injection its been twelve months now and I am walking with a limp, she said she would have a word with the doctor and to come back and see her in two weeks time.

I went back to mums and told her the CPN was going to ask the doctor if I could come off the Depixol injection, the next time I saw CPN again she told me that I could come off the injection and she asked me if I had anything to say, all I could think about at that time was I would not be able to go back to work, CPN also told me because things were not going to good at mums she would referrer me to the Grange Day Centre in Coalville.

In May 1996 I attended the grange day centre three times a week, started to feel better no suicidal thoughts just racing thoughts getting 6 hours a sleep a night and my life started to get better.

My benefits were seventy five pounds a week I had to pay fifteen pounds towards my divorce and give my mum twenty pounds a week board, I told my best friend that I needed to sell my car and get a cheaper one. One of my friends brought my car for one thousand five hundred so then I brought an older car for four hundred so I could survive. My divorce came through in August.

The social services sent for me to be means tested for Inca pacity benefit I had to Leicester to see one of their doctors and I passed..

Near to the end in August 1996 I applied for DLA benefit, my key worker at the grange day centre filled the form in for me. Four weeks later in September they awarded me middle rate for life. Then on the 15th of Oct I left mums house and went to live back in Ibstock in a bed-sit above a fish and chip shop.

## CHAPTER SIX

Back at Ibstock

It was a Saturday when I moved into my bed-sit, it all seemed so strange because I was sleeping in a cot room. All my friends went to a nightclub called Travellers Rest. I stayed in just realising where I was. My daughter only lived round the corner from me.

The week after I had to go and visit the Hawthorn centre to see my psychiatrist for the first time since I left the hospital. In my first consultation he asked me questions like.. How did I feel now that I had been taken off the injection? I told him that I couldn't sleep properly because of what has happened to me. All I wanted to ask him was, why was I given the injection? He replied I did not give it to you. I said to him you kept me on it whilst I was out in the community, then he couldn't answer me. He was only my out patients doctor. As I was on no medication he gave me Phenelzine tablets to take. I constantly took these tables for two weeks but they had loads of side effects to them. I couldn't breath very good and I started to gain weight.

My CPN had left so I had to see different CPN until I could get a regular one. I visited the Hawthorn Centre every month. I continued to go to the Grange day centre three times a week, my key worker moved from Nottingham to Ibstock so we started to see a lot more of each other. I started to visit her at home and have cups of tea with her. In December we started to have a relationship, she had two children from her previous relationship. Over Christmas the children had stayed with their father in Nottingham, so we spent Christmas together.

After New Years I would sleep three nights at her house and four nights at my bed-sit. I started to learn more about mental health as she knew a lot, and also about the mental health act 1983. She told me about Accuphase Clopixol and water, which is the doctor's strongest drug. It would knock you about for three days.

I changed my solicitors from Coalville to Ashby because my ex wife and me were arguing a lot about my shares in the house. We had a mortgage with Alliance and Leicester and the amalgamated with another bank; because my name was first on the mortgage I received a payment of One thousand two hundred pounds from the bank. The wife was not happy because I was given the money not her.

I continued seeing my daughter on a regular basis, as she only lived around the corner. I still continued to go to the Traveller Rest with my friends as I enjoyed dancing and listening to the music, it also helped keep me fit. As I wasn't taking any medication the mania set in and I began to get high and then the lows would come. I would have to stay in bed feeling Lethargic, Self-worthless and felling very sorry for myself, with very little sleep. I enjoyed feeling high at the time because it made me feel happy and my friends could see me happy and thought Jimmy's back to his old self. They didn't see the bad side of me.

I moved out of the cot room and went into a front room, which was bigger. I was getting income support because the bed-sit had all the other bills included. I had to pay my landlord twenty pounds a week. As the council wouldn't pay all the rent, not long after a flat across the road became empty, so I went to enquire about it and I moved in not long after. Which I felt happy about because I would have my own space again. I wouldn't have to share the kitchen or bathroom with anybody. I went to visit my mother every two weeks and I told her about the flat. I asked if I could have some furniture out of the club book for the flat. I applied for a Barclay card while I was living across the road in the bed-sit. I received one and I was given one thousand pound credit. The relationship with my key worker ended in July 1997.

My friend arranged his stag week away in Greece and I along with twenty six other lads went I had a nice time there getting away from everything, I started drinking a lot, I can remember lying on the beach on my back for six hours, my friend said you have not turned over. My thoughts were about my key worker. She realised that I didn't love her, as I just needed her in case I took ill again and I knew that she could get me out of hospital. Not long after I came back from Greece I had an appointment with my psychiatrist he was only a local doctor, I told him that I had been drinking again and that I was having episodes of highs and low and couldn't sleep properly because of what has happened. He replied I'm sorry but I cannot medicate you. I said your having a laugh aren't you; you're a psychiatrist why can't you help me? He told me that there were another psychiatrist starting at the Hawthorn Centre and that he will be my regular doctor. He would be able to help me. I left the Hawthorn Centre feeling very bitter and angry as I needed there help at this time.

I contacted an Advocacy worker to read my medical notes; I had to go to the Bradgate unit as by now Carlton-Hayes Hospital had closed down. My Advocacy worker, Psychiatrist and me were all present in the room to read my notes. I asked my Advocacy worker that my mother had said about me to the doctor went I was in hospital at Carlton-Hayes. Your mum said that you was doing okay she said. And what did my Ex wife say I asked, she just said that your marriage was all over. I asked the Psychiatrist why I was given the injection and he said you were diagnosed with paranoid schizophrenia. The advocacy worker told me to calm down. The psychiatrist said I am not your doctor I am retiring soon. When you try to take you life, you lost you insanity and the man above saved you, by then I knew that I had been wrongly diagnosed and my psychiatrist agreed with me. He said you should have never been given the injection. Then the Advocacy worker and me left the room. The Advocacy worker asked me if I was feeling all right to travel home on my own.

Instead of going home I went to see my mum. I told her that I had been wrongly diagnosed and that I had just been to the hospital to read my notes. Mum wasn't in a very good mood and said that I never should have had the relationship with my key worker. So then I went back to my flat. I got a letter through the post for me to go and see my new Consultant psychiatrist at the Hawthorn Centre, September 1997. My doctor and me had a long discussion about my past, he came across as a very good doctor, which I was glad to have him as my regular psychiatrist. I had a good half an hour with him I told him that I couldn't sleep properly because of what had happened in my past. He asked me to meet him again but this time I had to meet him at the brad gate unit to fill some forms in.

Two weeks later I went to the brad gate unit to have a consultation with my psychiatrist he asked me a lot of questions, because with him being my new doctor he wanted to get to know me better. I told him I took ill at thirty-three after I had answered all his questions and we had been chatting for a while he said do you know you have a mental illness? And I replied yes! He asked what medication could I give you? And I asked for Carbamazepine. He said might get a bad reaction. So I thought it would be best if I had a mood stabiliser. So then he said that we would try Lithium. He said that we would start you off on four hundred milligrams a day but you will have to have some blood test. After my blood tests had come through he put my tablets up to six hundred milligrams daily. I changed my GP'S from Whitwick to a surgery in Coalville.

In November I started doing voluntary work for the Befriending Scheme. You had to go on a nine weeks course; after I had past my course I started to help other people with mental health problems. I would take them out for a game of pool or go and visit them at home and listen to their problems. Which I hoped it would do them good as well as me.

Christmas was here again I spend most of it down my mother's house, as I didn't want to be on my own. For the New Year I stayed at my flat and didn't go out. My key worker rang me and asked me if I went out anywhere and I told her that I stayed in my flat. She said that I stopped at your friends for the night. I put the phone down on her as I thought she was just trying to screw my head up and come between my friends and me. I stopped going down the Travellers Rest because she still went there. I made some new friends one of which lived above the fish shop where I used to live. The other one lived at the other end of Ibstock. We started to go down Jimmy Dean's nightclub, taking Lithium made me very thirsty so I drank a lot of beer and didn't get drunk. My other friend was an ex minor like me and he was also going through a divorce. I invited him around my flat and we went out on a regular basis for a drink in Whitwick. While we were out drinking he asked me if I fancied going to Newcastle with him as he had friends down there.

June 1998, I went with him to Newcastle we had a good time it was one big piss up. His friends were also very friendly. We only stayed there for two nights and then travelled back home. The next time we went out for a drink down Whitwick some of the lads were talking about going to Blackpool for a stag weekend and asked me if I wanted to go along with them. In July we went to Blackpool we started drinking at eleven in the morning at the Pleasure beach. We stopped drinking at seven and went for a shower then we went back out to the tower lounge and onto a nightclub. We stopped drinking at two in the morning I had spend ninety pound on drink and was still standing, I just couldn't get drunk on Lithium. I just slurred my words. I had lost my friends but I had a card on me with the bed and breakfast address on it. So I showed it to the taxi driver and asked him to take me there. The next day I didn't drink much we just went sight seeing and travelled home the day after. The following weekend my two friends and me went out for a drink where we normally went and went on to Jimmy Dean's I didn't feel very well that night and I got back to my flat. I didn't sleep very well, my head was pounding it was worse than a hangover. I thought I was going mental again. All Sunday I was still in pain and didn't go out I couldn't wait until Monday morning to ring up my CPN at the Hawthorn Centre. I told her I wasn't feeling very well and she said do you want to come down and see the doctor? Or do you want the doctor to come and see you at home? I went straight to see the doctor. I told the doctor that I had been drinking heavily and my head was so sore more than just a hangover. He asked me if I would like to go into hospital just for two weeks and I said yes! I went back to my flat and packed a bag then I rang my mum and explained what I was doing. She told me not to go in there; I didn't tell her that I thought my drink had been spiked! I rang a taxi up and they took me to the brad gate unit when I arrived at the main entrance they told me to follow the signs to Ashby ward. I felt scared and all alone. I didn't really want to open the door because I didn't know how long I would be in for before I got back out.

I walked through Ashby ward doors. The first person I saw was the ward manager who used to work at Carlton-Hayes Hospital. He said we have a bed ready for you Jimmy. I also saw two other nurses from Carlton-Hayes. They showed me to my dormitory. I unpacked my bag and went and sat in the television room.

A student doctor came and asked me some questions I told him that I wasn't feeling very well, that my head was spinning and I had had no sleep for two days. Shortly after, my psychiatrist wanted to see me there wasn't many people in with the doctor, he asked me some questions. I told the doctor that I thought that I had my drink spiked and he said that he would get me a urine sample done. On the Wednesday it was ward round there were a lot of people in with the doctor I asked the doctor if my drink had been spiked and he didn't answer me. He just told me to stay in hospital another week. I understood why he wouldn't tell me in case I went out of hospital and did something, which I would regret later. Even the nurses on the ward wouldn't tell me anything. I didn't like the atmosphere I was in, it was a completely different hospital compared to Carlton-Hayes there were more beds in the dormitory and not a lot of privacy. Some patients had there own rooms, there was a court yard were the nurses would let you out for a walk until the doctor let you go out on your own. The courtyard was in between the hospital corridors and the ward, so that the nurses could keep an eye on you out of their office windows. As I was a voluntary patient I was allowed to walk around the grounds and then go back onto the ward.

On Friday I left the Bradgate Unit and went home. I contact the Christian care and counselling as I thought I needed help. I began my counselling it would take about four weeks. In between I met a woman who worked at the fish shop across the road from where I lived. At first we were just friends (Then later on in life we married). I felt like I needed a short break so I went away for two days on my own to Matlock bath. The first night was okay after breakfast I took a walk along lovers' lane and went up on top of the hill. I felt something was over powering me. My head was telling me to go to the edge of the cliff I looked down and I was only was a foot away from the cliff edge I was so scared I had trouble with drawing myself back off the cliff edge. As my brain was telling me to go off the cliff. I managed to get myself back onto the path and get back down to the bottom I went back to my bed and breakfast and had a shower. After my shower I lay on the bed and started to relax I closed my eyes and felt my self drifting slowly down to the bottom of the cliff and slowly drifting back up. Which went on for an hour I managed to bring myself round. I went out for a drink at seven o'clock I had four pints at the Fishpond then went to leave the pub. As I came out I felt like I'd gone back in time. I went to another pub called the Midland inn I just had one pint in there then went to the toilet. When I went into the toilet the pub was full when I came out it was empty. Everybody had left to catch the last train back home. I felt like this was my journey to my bi-polar disorder.

The next day I went back home my psychiatrist came to my flat with my CPN. I let them in, my doctor wanted me to go back into hospital I told him no, as I didn't want to tell him that I was having counselling. So the doctor gave me some extra medication it was ten mg of Olanzapine. A week later the doctor and my CPN came back to visit me at my flat but I wouldn't let them in because I only had one week left to do with my counsellor. At my last counselling session the lady told me to go to church and that God would want me to forgive my mother. I went back home I made an appointment to go to church. When I went to church I prayed if I had to go back into hospital it would be a place of safety for me and I also forgave my mother and drank some Holy water.

I went back to my flat not long after the phone rang it was my best friend telling me to stay away form the ex miner because he was the one that had spiked my drink I told him I knew myself as it could only been two people. I didn't have a car at the time I knew he would be on the afternoon shift so at half past one I got on my bike with my baseball bat down my coat I had no intention of using it but I knew he was my enemy and I just wanted to scare him so he would leave me alone as I was on my bike making my way to where he worked he over took me in his car when I arrived at the car park I got off my bike and made my way through the shop floor with the baseball bat still in my coat. I thought I was Grant Mitchell he was in the canteen I shouted him and let him see the baseball bat he came towards me and I marched him back through the shop floor and to the entrance of his work place. His work friend was with him I told him if he ever done anything like that again to me I would come to his house and use it. He didn't say a word he looked scared and I felt that I had scared him off for good. I got back on my bike and went home.

On Saturday morning I went down Coalville and drew all the money out of my bank account. All that was left in there was a penny. I went and had my haircut really short then went into a shop and brought a suit and an orange tie. I also brought a pair of shoes that was one size to big for me. I went back to my flat and tried my suit on I thought I was Grant Mitchell. I went out that night to The Boot for a drink I had my new suit, shoes and sunglasses on. I sat on the stool at the bar drinking my pint and my best friend came in and sat next to me. I said 'How are you mate' and he didn't recognise me. I said you have known me for eight years and I kicked his stool and it scared him. He knew who I was then but he still couldn't say anything to me because I had had my haircut really short and had a goatee beard. I went into the toilets where I saw another one of my close friends and I asked him if he had slept with my key worker on New Years Eve. He went on to tell me that she slept on his sofa and I said that I would forgive him and walked out. I felt so good about myself as the highs had started to kick in, so I thought to myself that I would go in The Ram for a pint before I went home. I felt like people were whispering about me, I had a game of pool and I don't know what came over me but I through two pool balls behind the bar and then left. I got back in my flat; I was so high there was no way that I was going to sleep. I lay on the bed I had racing thoughts that I was going to be the king of Scotland. If I didn't get out of Ibstock soon a laser gun would shoot me. I thought that I was invisible that only a laser gun could kill me. I got it into my head that a limo was going to pick me up at six o'clock in the morning I started ducking and diving under my window. I thought that on the horizon out of my window that there would be a sniper trying to kill me.

I started to empty my flat carrying everything outside and putting most of it into a skip which was outside my flat. I even picked up the fridge freezer and it felt like I was just picking up a shopping bag. I lay back on my bed all I could think about was that I was going to become the king of Scotland and all the ex-miners would line the streets and the police would be at junction twenty-three to see me off in my limo.

Six o'clock came I left four hundred and twenty pounds on my kitchen table. I got a sports bag and put my miner's lamp and plates, photos of my father and one or two of my personal things in it. Then I put the bag in the dustbin, which with my head being in a mess I was meant to be taking them with me. I started to get worked up and worried that the limo wasn't coming, I knew I needed professional help and didn't know what to do because it was a Sunday morning. I knew I had to do something wrong to get me back into a psychiatric hospital. I went to the skip and picked out some house bricks and went down the drive crossed the road and smashed the fish shop windows. I was so high the brick just felt like boxes of matches. The fish shop owner came to talk to me he asked me why I had done this and I told him I was half Greek and half Scottish. Whilst we were talking the police arrived and they took me away to Loughborough police station. I told the police I had left four hundred and twenty pounds on my kitchen table but they just carried onto the station. After we had arrived they took some photos of me and put me in a cell. This was the first time I had ever been in a police cell in my life. The police kept opening and closing the shutter every fifteen minuets. They gave me something to eat it was fish and chips.

Monday afternoon I had to see the police doctor, he asked me some questions. I told him that I was going to be king of Scotland and that the limo was waiting outside the police station for me to take me to Scotland. After a few more questions the doctor left the room and when he returned he informed me that my doctor wanted to see me from the Bradgate Unit. They handcuffed me and put me in the back of the police car. I didn't mention anything in the car until I reached the entrance of the Bradgate Unit. I thanked them for bringing me to a place of safety the policemen took my handcuffs off and took me to the Ashby ward.

## CHAPTER SEVEN

I thought I was the king of Scotland

October 4th 1998, the nurses checked my pockets and told me to go and sit down. I thought straight away that I was a detained prisoner. Only half an hour later I looked around and saw eight nurses coming towards me, they got hold of me and took me to my bed. They didn't tell me what they were doing to me; they pulled down my trousers and injected me. When I came round I got out of my bed looked into the mirror and I had a lot of stubble and I realised that I needed a shave.  I asked another patient how long have I been there? He said that I had been asleep for three days, then I realised that I had been given Accuphase. I went to the nurse's office and asked them for a razor, some shaving foam and some soap. As when I arrived at the hospital I did not have any belongings with me. The nurse told me that it would be ward round and if I would be all right to see the doctor? I replied yes as soon as I have cleaned myself up.

I went in to see the doctor and he asked me how I was? I said that I have had a good sleep doctor! It has just left me with a headache. He asked me why I smashed the Chip shop windows? I told him that I didn't know what came over me but I can tell you something I'm going to be the King of Scotland! Are you? What makes you think that? I told him that I was half Scottish and half

Greek I wouldn't tell him any more. So I asked him if I could leave ward round?
The nurses told me that I could only go around the courtyard with supervision. I asked how I was going to get any money? Not until the doctor says that you can go out of the hospital and be able to get to the bank, as my benefits are paid into the bank. I asked the nurse if I could borrow some money for the drinks machine. It was just outside Ashby ward doors, whilst I was getting my drink I saw the police bringing another patient in. he didn't want to go through the doors I told him that it would be better for him to go through the easy way as they will Accuphase you. Then after that we became friends, he walked in with his suit on just like me, and he was a fellow Scotchman just like me.

I told him how I ended up there and I thought that I was going to be the King of Scotland. He said you better know who your friends are we were both high laughing and joking in the smoke room. It was getting me down not being able to have any change of clothing, my benefits were paid into the bank but my doctor wouldn't let me off the ward because he knew that I was still high and ill.

The nurse told me that I had been sectioned two I just managed to appeal in time with in the fourteen days of my tribunal. The

Doctor let me go to Ibstock with a nurse because he wanted me to know and see what I had done to my flat now that I was in a reasonable frame of mind. I picked up some clothing and went to the bank to get some money. I also went in Coalville to buy a Walkman stereo then went back into the hospital. I went into the smoke room and I had never smoked before in my life and I lit up a king Edward cigar, I felt that this was part of my bi-polar disorder and still felt high. I went for a walk around the courtyard listened to my music which would make me more higher. I was listening to only the strong survive by Billy Paul. I'd do two hundred laps around the courtyard, when I returned back onto the ward a nurse pinned me down marched me into seclusion, turned my face down onto the mattress took of my clothes apart from my boxer shorts and then injected me with Accuphase. They slammed the doors behind them.

It was scary being in seclusion for the first time knowing that you cant get out.

I just covered myself over with the blanket and I had fast racing thoughts in my head and also a sore head, it felt like a giant hangover. I had half hour sleep in there, three hours later the nurses let me out. I had to go and see the doctor again in ward round. I asked him why have I been given Accuphase again? He didn't answer me. He told me that they had to change my medication to four hundred milligrams of Lithium and four hundred milligrams of Quetiapine. Two days later I had an argument with the nurse about my medication they told me that I had taken it, I told them that I hadn't. I kicked him in the leg and then ran out to the courtyard. The nurses wouldn't come out to me, I went back into the medication room started to argue with the nurses again, then a nurses gave me a rugby tackle pinned me down to the floor. There were six to eight of them. They put me into the seclusion room. They took all my clothes of apart form my underwear, lay me flat down on the bed and injected me with Accuphase, they also gave me another injection I asked them what it was, they said it was Haloperidol. It calmed me down then they left the room, they kept me in for a good six hours before they let me out.

My friend asked me if I was okay. We went into the smoke room and I lit up a cigar, there was another Scotsman in the smoke room we had a great laugh.    I was allowed of the ward for a walk. I found myself on the helicopter pad at Glenfied hospital. Singing only the strong survive high as a kite went back onto the ward and told a nurse what I had done. She didn't half look funny at me. The nurses grabbed hold of me again and took me into the seclusion room and gave me Accuphase again. I stood up on the bed and burst out laughing and told them that there strongest drug didn't have any effect on me any more. There were a lot of nurses in the room I told them that they were all vampires then they locked the door. When I was in the room I just stayed awake and kept walking round in circles. Three hours later they let me out. I went straight into the smoke room once again and lit up a cigar. Talking to my friend and the other Scotsman I told them that I was going to be the king of Scotland they started to talk about all the kings of Scotland. The other Scotsman knew so much about the other kings of Scotland. Then it started to worry me I didn't want to learn anymore it made me even higher having these beliefs. I started to listen to century radio until two o'clock in the morning I went into the

Scotsman's bedroom and tipped him out of bed. The bed felt so light then I went back into my bedroom. He told the nurses what I had done to him after breakfast I apologised to him and told him that I was sorry for what I had done. I sat in the living room for a while, and then a nurse came to me and said that I would have to be given Accuphase. I asked what again? I haven't done anything wrong! The doctor said that you have got to so I let them Accuphase me again.

I went to bed that night and started to feel restless and agitated and I couldn't sleep so I went and told the nurse how I was feeling he said that he would give me some diazepam to help me relax and sleep. I woke up the next morning for breakfast I went out into the courtyard I walked around fifty times then stopped for a cigar, then I would do another fifty laps listening to my music only the strong survive. I went back onto the ward and had my dinner then went back out to the courtyard again and did another fifty laps the nurses were watching me from there office tears running down my face I was feeling high by then it just was starting to get dark. By the time I went back onto the ward I had walked four hundred times around the courtyard. A nurse came over to me and told me that they were going to Accuphase me again they said that they would put me to sleep this time by giving me two hundred milligrams. After they had injected me I asked the nurse if they would get me a drink of pop. As my throat was getting dry. I lay back down onto the bed I had racing thoughts going through my head. My head was spinning I had to take the thoughts from the front of my head slowly to the back as I wanted to get out of the bed but I was taking my thoughts from the front to the back of my mind too quickly. I stood up and fell back into the bed there was a fine art to it after about an hour I got out of the bed.

The duty doctor wanted to see me he said to me do you realised that you have just been given Accuphase? I replied yes doctor but my words were slurry he asked me some more questions but I couldn't remember. I went back onto the ward I knew that I had to keep myself on the ward and not to go back to my bedroom as I felt that I would have been in my bed for a long while.

I hope I have explained the best way as I can about having two hundred milligrams of Accuphase. After dinner I went to the vending machine and started drinking Pepsi max. At ten o'clock I went for my medication, I knew I was in the Looney bin but it just felt as though I was in a desert. I was so thirsty I had drunk twenty cans of Pepsi max. The nurses came into the smoke room to have a look around and my empty cans were all over the windowsill. I asked the night nurse why was I given two hundred milligrams of Accuphase, she said it was because I am a big bloke. I knew myself your only suppose to have one hundred and fifty milligrams. It took me three days to shake the Accuphase out of my system, drinking all that Pepsi max. I felt like I had flushed all the bad shit out. After breakfast I went to the nurses office and asked if I could have some money out of the safe. My flat key was in there and I took it without the nurse seeing. Later in the afternoon I took a walk around the grounds and the mania was starting to kick in again I was having elevations of excitement and I felt good inside. I walked across the A50 outside the hospital grounds this was a massive high. I ran down to county halls roundabout crossed over there and stopped at the petrol station I had a thick brown leather coat on and I stopped and thought to myself why aren't I sweating after running so fast? I started to run again to Markfield village laughing to myself I thought I was the bionic man. I turned around and there was the double Decker bus, I got on the bus and I couldn't believe who I saw. It was my brother in law driving the bus. I said I haven't got any small change mate and he said go and sit down upstairs. He knew where I had come from!

I got off the bus at Coalville and caught another bus to Ibstock and went to my flat. I thought to myself I am enjoying these highs; I have never experienced anything like this in my life. I got onto my bike and went up Common hill. I looked down at my gears and I was only in fifth gear. It was so easy going up the hill, I had so much energy and I thought that I was E.T. I came back down the hill and decided to go up some more hills. After a while I went back to my flat and I went back out again and brought some fish and chips. It was getting late, I went back to my flat and not long after the police came to my door and said that they had come to take me back to the hospital. On the way back to the hospital I told the police when I get out of hospital I am going to be the King of Scotland and save the world. They kept a straight face and took me to the entrance of the Bradgate

# I THOUGHT I WAS THE KING OF SCOTLAND

Unit. Not long after I was back on the ward the vampires came for me I knew what they were going to do, they came from all different wards. I ran into seclusion myself took my clothes of apart from my underwear and I told them that they better not give me two hundred milligrams. At this time I was getting angry I let them give me the injection, I stood back upon to the bed and burst out laughing at them. I told them that they were all wankers; they were all standing around me in a circle. The room was full of vampires I burst out laughing again. They just stood there in amazement then they walked out and closed the door behind them. Six hours later they let me out. Two days later I had to see me psychiatrist he asked me why I escaped? I said that the mania had set in again I was that high I was running that fast that I could keep up with the cars I was over exaggerating and if didn't do myself any favours. The doctor gave me some extra medication, five milligrams of diazepam three times a day to shut me down. I got section three for that I lost all of my privileges with in a week the diazepam was shutting me down. I asked the nurses if I could appeal against my section three they said it would have to go to a mental health review tribunal. It would take up to six to eight weeks for me to see a solicitor. I knew that I had to behave myself from now on, not to bother any of the patients or nurses keeping myself clean, eating their food and talking to the other patients. My two fellow Scots men where still in here I couldn't watch telly. I asked the nurses if I could always have my own room, as I didn't want to go back into the dormitory with it being so noisy and just a curtain away from another patient. As I was in there for sleep. They gave me my own room with a toilet I told the nurses I would be able to settle down now and that would have been my last Accuphase. The nurses told me that they have been in contact with my mother and she said that she didn't want to visit me. So I rang a friend Janet from the Fish Shop and I also rang my daughter up, as I hadn't seen her for six weeks. My daughter came first to see me, my ex wife brought her. I had my suit on and my daughter didn't recognise me. We asked the nurse if it was okay to go to the hospital shop and nurse said yes! They didn't stop very long. A couple of days later Janet came to visit me I told her that I had made a mess of the flat and could we still be friends? I gave her the key to my flat and asked her if she would sort it out for me and to put the key under the old fridge outside my flat. When Janet left I went into the smoke room I felt at least I have got one friend and that's all you need to believe in you.

It was ward round the next day my friend and me put our suits on so we would look smart for the doctor. I didn't realise it wasn't doing me any favours because I felt good when I was wearing my suit. I was in more control of myself I could see there were a lot of people in the room. The doctor said that he would keep me on the same medication, as it seemed to be working for me. I went back to my bedroom and changed my clothes. I asked the nurses if I had any of my privileges back? Only escorted walks round the courtyard for fifteen minutes. I stopped my singing, which I am a crap singer anyway. My appeal date came through in December my solicitor came to see me on the ward, he said that we might not be able to lift your section three but we may be able to get the doctor to let you have leave slowly and that's what happened.

On the fifteenth of December I was given an over night stay to see if I could cope on my own.

I knew I was on my way out. The doctor asked me how I had coped. He said I will give you some more leave at the weekend and I handled that okay. I had a week off over Christmas and the New Year spending some of the time at my mothers. I went back to hospital after the New Year and in my thoughts I was thinking back to last year and what a year it had been! And I never wanted to go through that again. I lit a cigar up the diazepam was having more effect on me. I knew when I had to see the doctor again that I would ask him to take me off the morning tablet because I was feeling lethargic. He continued to give me zopilone for my sleep. I also stayed on four hundred milligrams of lithium and four hundred milligrams of Quetiapine. My friend was due to leave I told him that we would stay in contact and meet up when I get out. I felt all-alone then I got more leave on a section 117. The nurses' saw I was doing well on my leave and feeling a lot better. So the next time I went into ward round the doctor said the nurses have told me how well you have progressed and that he was going to lift the section. I was free to go home after spending twenty-two weeks in hospital.

I arrived back home; my friend Janet had made a good job of my flat. I had lots of mail to open; I knew the first thing I had to do was to claim my benefits back. There was a letter from the council telling me because I had been in hospital for quite a while they had stopped paying my rent to the landlord. So that meant that I was in rent arrears of two months. The landlord came to see me with the bill this was enough to put me back into hospital I felt like I had had a big weight on my shoulders. The landlord was only across the road I asked him if I could pay it back by giving five or ten pounds a week. He was a good understanding landlord and he let me off with the rent arrears. I went up to the co-op supermarket to do some shopping, my basket was full I felt agitated. Everybody around me looked so calm it looked easy for them queuing at the tills. I dropped my basket and ran out of the shop. I knew I would have to go back at some point when the shop wasn't that busy.

The first few weeks of leaving hospital I found hard coping on my own, my best friend came to visit me we had a long chat. He told me that his other friends had told him to stay away from me else they wouldn't talk to him again. He said that he was sorry and then he left. How I look at it first time in hospital it could happen to anyone, second times in hospital people are weary of you and the third time you are the village nutter. I had a lot of people crossing the road and they wouldn't stop and talk to me they would look the other way but I got used to that after a while. Janet came around to visit me before she went to work, we had a cup of tea and she told me that we would always be friends. I asked her if I could take her out for a drink, then after a month we started a relationship. Every month the CPN would come to visit me, my psychiatrist wanted to see me every month. The five months of my life went by I felt as my medication wasn't working anymore and I was heading for another break down. Me and Janet were looking forward to a short break at Matlock it was the first week in September I had racing thoughts going through my head and my sleep pattern was all over the place. On Friday I told Janet to have the weekend to get all her jobs done because we was going away on Monday. I didn't want her to know I wasn't very well. Friday lunchtime my CPN came to visit me I was wearing my suit and I told her that I was going to Coalville. She asked me if she could have my mobile number she gave me a lift to Ravenstone. I just got to Coalville and my mobile rang it was my CPN she said that the doctor wanted to see me. I told her that I didn't want to see him. So then I switched my phone off.

Over the weekend I didn't get any sleep at all, I was agitated I though something was going to happen to me but I didn't want to let Janet down. Sunday came I went out for a long walk and I started walking like a soldier, quite fast. This scared me at the time, I got back into my flat, later that night I rang Janet and told her that I couldn't find the train tickets and that I had put her spending money on the kitchen table. When Janet came down the next day we were suppose to be going to Matlock for a few days. We arrived at

Loughborough train station. We got onto the train to Derby then I started acting strange when we arrived at Derby, station I got my bag left Janet and got on the wrong train. I felt guilty that I had left Janet at Derby train station. I asked the woman on the train where the train was going she said to London. I had a cross in my pocket and I got it out I told her to stop the train she said the train will be stopped at Leicester train station. I got off the train at Leicester went into the toilets put my suit on and left my bag in the toilet the mania had started to kick in again I thought that I was invisible. I walked down to Charles street went into Willie Thorns snooker hall the last time I was in there I was only eighteen.

I asked for a pint of milk and paid with a twenty-pound note and told her to keep the change I had three hundred and fifty pounds on me and I felt as if I was a millionaire. I had a pint of lager which I again paid with a twenty pound note and again told her to keep the change. I put twenty pound into the bandit a bloke said to me that I wasn't playing it properly I said you play it then, he said what if I win? I told him if he won he could keep the money, I had another pint of lager and told the bar staff the keep the change again. Then I asked a bloke if he wanted a game of snooker for money? I had three games for twenty pound I lost all three I hadn't picked a queue up for years. I only watched it on TV. He said to me that I was playing the right shots but the balls weren't going into the pockets. I asked him if he wanted to play double or quits if I lost I would give him hundred and twenty pounds. I lost that game and I gave him the money. What money I had left I tried to give it away to this couple who had been watching us playing snooker but they wouldn't take it off me. I had over a hundred pounds left so I flushed it down the toilet as I thought I was going to be the king of Scotland and I wouldn't need any English money.

Then I went and sat down next to the bar. The bloke who I played snooker with said we know you're a millionaire. I said Stephen Henry is going to pick me up he looked at me and went up to one of the ladies behind the bar then came back over to me and said Stephen Henrys not coming for you. I thought shit what am I going to do now? I got no money I waited until six o'clock and then I left I thought If I walked around Leicester all day and all night and follow the yellow lines I would be fit to be the king of Scotland. I can remember standing outside the holiday inn and Janet' mum rang my mobile on the phone it said mum and I thought that it was my mum ringing. So I chucked the phone away by then the time was getting on I have never heard voices before in my life. A old friend of mine called Cue was killed in a car accident on the way to work one morning I was standing at the church doors where he got married and I shouted Cue and he shouted back Jimmy. I was banging on the church doors for a while trying to get in then I left and started marching like a soldier I sat down near some railings people were coming out of a night club.

I was hallucinating and having dilutions bright lights were coming up close to me and going away again some of the people threw some money at me I told them I wasn't a tramp. I started to walk away again following the yellow lines I wished I had picked up the money now because I was starting to dehydrate. I found myself in dead ends and found it hard to get out. Morning came this felt so strange I had been walking all day and to see the day light coming I looked up and seen a pub. A woman was hanging out of the window watering the hanging baskets I took my jacket off and stood under the dripping water. That felt so good at the time. The landlord came out and gave me a cup of tea after half an hour he told me to leave. I didn't follow the yellow lines anymore I just started walking I found myself in the town centre. I felt like I was in hell, the mental pain I was experiencing only a fellow sufferer or a specialist would understand how I felt.

 I was getting so worried that I wasn't going to be the king of Scotland.

## CHAPTER EIGHT

## Stop The Old Bill

As I was walking along passed St Margate bus station I sat down near a small wall. I took off my shoes and socks my feet were covered in blisters. I was in so much physical and mental pain I didn't know what to do, I walked along to a set of traffic lights and a police car was there, I banged my fist on the window and said you've got to take me to a mental hospital. Bradgate Unit, he told me to get into the back of the car and stay there. The policeman got out of his car and talked on his phone to his other colleges and explained to them that he has a Schizophrenic in the back of his car. The policeman took me to the police station on they way I told him that I was going to be king of Scotland. It was only a small police station that we arrived at; the officers asked me what I had done to myself. I told them that I had spent all day and all night following the yellow lines all the way around Leicester. They got me a bowl of water so that I could bathe my feet and some water for me to drink. They also gave me some sandwiches. They asked me who my next of kin was, I was that ill I'd gone back in time and thought I was still with my ex wife so I gave them her number. The police officer came back to me and told me that my psychiatrist wanted to see me. I thought to myself at least I haven't got to go through police doctors, so I let them take me to the Brad Gate Unit. I handled walking onto the ward out of my own free will, I told the nurses what I had done. I also told the nurse that I had left my bag at the train station toilets and also that I had left my girlfriend Janet at Derby train station. The nurses were very good with me, one of the male nurses was a nurse on the old ward at Carton-Hayes Hospital, and he bandaged my feet up because a lot of my skin had gone of the pads of my feet. The next day came they gave me a wheel chair it was hard to get my breakfast in a wheel chair and getting used to how to push it around the ward.

It was Wednesday and it was ward round I went in to see the doctor, they had moved the furniture around for me so that I could get in with my wheel chair. I told the doctor that I thought I was going to be the king of Scotland. I also told him that my dad had sent me some special shoes that had a magnet in the heel so that I could follow all the yellow lines all the way around Leicester and if I succeeded I was fit enough to be the king. The doctor replied you have been through hell and back, he took me off my current medication and all he could give me was painkillers and told me to keep bathing my feet until the skin grew back. I knew I was still in hell and it's not a very nice place to be. I went to get some dinner still finding it hard to get around in my wheel chair, but the nurses just let my get on with it. After a couple of days I was getting in and out the toilet fine and getting myself in a nice hot bath. I knew it was going to be along time to get my feet better and my mental health state.

# I THOUGHT I WAS THE KING OF SCOTLAND

I got Janet to come in and visit me I told her how very sorry I was for leaving her. She couldn't believe the state of my feet. I didn't want Janet to see me like this I was horrible to her and told her to go and not to come and see me until I was out of the wheelchair and my mental health was better. I can remember being in the smoke room in my wheelchair understanding people who couldn't walk I felt disabled at both ends. It took me two weeks to get out of that wheelchair I got a section two and I told the doctor when I get out of here I want to be king of Scotland and that I would have to do ten years in and out of a psychiatric hospital. (It took me to my next breakdown to explain everything to the doctor about all these thought that came into my head).

Janet came to visit me again I was fine with her this time, she went and got me a bowl of water so that I could bathe my feet in it. Janet would come and visit me everyday and stay on the ward with me for four to five hours at a time. Coming off my Quetiapine and lithium I sat in the smoke room and I had my hands on the arm of the chair. I got an electric shook in both of my thumbs. I looked up to the sky and I thought the world was turning around that Scotland was becoming England and vies versa. I thought that the patients in the smoke room were going to crown me the king. I knew this was sheer madness but I was still living in hell. I went in ward round again to see the doctor and her told me that he cannot give me any medication just yet, I told the doctor that I wanted to leave and get out of the hospital. I knew that my section two was going to head onto a section three. He said to me your going nowhere so I stormed out of ward round angry. I was kicking all the doors on the ward the nurses took me into a room and Accuphase me. I told the nurses all I wanted was peace in my life and they said we do too. I knew by then that my doctor was my enemy after being Accuphase I walked into the toilet and the lights were flashing on and off I thought I was committing to god and talking to him. One of the nurses came down to me and said what are you doing talking to yourself? I told him that I was talking to god. I went for a walk around the courtyard and went by an orange light and started to talk to it thinking that god had turned it off when I had spoken to it and then the light would come back on. I knew that I had to hold on to my Christian faith. Faith came first then love but hope was not coming my way. The next time at ward round when I seen the doctor he asked my why I was talking to the lights in the toilets? I told him all there was to do in this hospital was to smoke and talk to god I told the doctor that I wanted to get out. The next day I saw the doctor in the nurses office I told him that he wanted to keep me here for the rest of my life and that he was a crap doctor and that he thought that he was a god on to his own. I went back into my bedroom to calm down fifteen minutes later four nurses came into my bedroom pulled my trousers down and Accuphase me. Not long after that I started to feel unwell I was sweating; I had muscle stiffness and paranoid behaviour. I was looking at the light in my bedroom I switched the light on I had a vision in my head that the light would beam up and take me into heaven this felt like hell at the time. I was bending over backwards and forwards on the bed trying to catch my breath I thought I was going to die. This was like something out of the exorcists this was going on for a long while it felt like it was never going to end then the nurses came into my bedroom. I can't remember a lot after that but they wheeled me out of the Ashby ward and onto a ward in the Glenfied hospital. This was to find out what was wrong with me, I had trouble breathing this went on for a long while I thought it was fifty fifty, whether I was going to live or die. It was a painful and frightening experience I can remember Janet being at the side of me I knew I had to be strong to fight this and had to will to live as the nurse just couldn't do anything for me it was just a matter of time. After a while my breathing returned to normal and they took me back to my room.

They found out what had caused the seizures I had Neurleptic Malignant syndrome due to antipsychiotic drugs which now I know I'm very sensitive to most of them, I cannot have any more Accuphase ever again. Neurleptic Malignant syndrome rare and life threatening disorder most often caused by an adverse reaction to antipsychotic drugs. My symptoms were high fever, sweating, unstable blood pressure, paranoia behaviour and a high blood count.

The nurses had to keep a regular check on my blood pressure and to take my blood to check the count levels. I'm so glad that the nurse found me when he did or I believe I wouldn't be here today to tell the storey. There are some good nurses on the Ashby ward. It was coming up to the end of my section two I refused any medication that they wanted to give me I told them that it was not agreeing with me anymore. It was the first week in October 1999, Janet came to visit me she brought us both some lunch the weather was nice so we went out into the courtyard to eat it, after lunch we went for a walk round the courtyard then I just stopped in the middle of the grass looked up at the sky and started singing the Light house family to god by then I was getting higher and higher I thought I was in the garden of Eden and that I was singing to god. The nurses were watching me through their office window Janet just sat on the bench while I was singing to god I thought I had special powers and that I was communicating with god, the nurse came out to speak to me he asked me if I would go back onto the ward as the nurses wanted to talk to me. When I went back onto the ward and into my bedroom the nurses came in to talk to me and they asked Janet if she would leave the room, they told me that I had to go into ITU unit belvoir ward as you need one to one care and we are not able to give you the care you need over here the nurse told me to pack my things and then four nurses escorted me over there.

Before I go on about my illness I would like to explain a bit about the lay out of the ward or prison I was now in, as you looked at the building from the out side all the windows were tinted grass so when people walked by they could not see in, as you got to the front entrance there were two double doors which were locked at all times and you had to speak through an intercom to be let in, just in side was a waiting area with some tables and chairs and a toilet, then before you went onto the ward there was another locked door which you had to wait at to be let onto the ward and if you had any visitors they had a little glass hatch with sliding doors were you had to hand over all your belonging as you were not allowed any thing on the ward it was just like visiting some one in prison the only difference was you did get searched before you went on the ward. There were ten members of staff and eight patients, to the left of the ward which I called the left wing were ten bedrooms every patient had there own bedroom and it had a small TV room the room next to that was a small office used for ward rounds they was a quit room and the nurses office was in the middle of the ward with glass windows which I used to call the goal fish bowl, so they could see what the patients were doing, a games room and another big TV room where the nurses went for a smoke there was a door leading out side to a small courtyard where you could go for fifth teen minutes everyday for escorted with a nurse, there was one toilet and a bathroom and a canteen. On the right side of the ward were the seclusion area with servile seclusion room and one big shower room.

When I got onto the ward they kept all my belonging apart from my clothes. The first night you had to sleep in seclusion with the door open it was to get the feel of the place and the different surrounding I could not sleep so I went for a look around the seclusion area but they told me to go back into seclusion and get some sleep, morning came the nurse told me after lunch they were going to give me my own bedroom but when my visitors came they were not allowed in there, you had to cue up to get into the canteen for your meals the nurse would unlock the door then give you your knife and fork after you finished eating you would have to give your knife and fork back to the nurse before you left the room and the nurse would lock the door again until next meal time, I thought to myself this is like a prison that they just gave you medication and the nurses were wardens one of the nurses held me say they were wardens and he said you do not look at us like that do you? I just smiled at him and walked away I felt safe in because there were no vampires, I knew if you were going to blow they would just put you in seclusion and not give you any needles. Lather that day I got my own room it was very posh I even had desk and a chair and my own wash room with a toilet if there was not so many restrictions on the ward this would be a four star hotel, I put my cloths away and then I went for a look round, there was a vending machine which you could have free drinks and a payphone. I went to ask the nurse for my razor and toiletries he gave me a peace of foil and some blue tac so I could stick the foil on the wall as there was not any mirrors on the wall after you had finished you had to give your things back to the nurse, it was hard work not being very well to survive in here some of the patients would not talk, it was tense you did not know whether there was going to be a fright or not. The trolley man only came once a day and he was not allowed on the ward so you had to tell the nurses what you wanted and they would get it for you, they had two wards rounds a week one on a Tuesday afternoon and one on a Friday, the visiting times were also different you were only allowed on the ward at visiting times which were two hours in the afternoon and two hours at night. Wednesday morning not feeling very well and also feeling a bit high I was finding it hard to cope, later that day I played a game of pool with the nurses I was getting on well with these nurses I was feeling comfortable with them we started laughing and joking, I could not settle or sleep with me being high the next couple of days went by in a blur me trying to get use to these different surrounding. Friday came it was ward round and I went in to see the doctor, I told the doctor that I was going to be the King of Scotland and that my helicopter was waiting outside for me for when I got out of here, the doctor laughed my other doctor always kept a straight face when I told him these things I knew I was not going to be the king I just had a laugh with the doctor, they told me later that day I would have to have my tribunal the date was set for next Friday I can not really remember much has I was to ill and at this stage not sleeping at night at all the days just became a blur to me all I do was just listen to my music, the nurses told me that tomorrow was my tribunal I asked Janet if she would come to the tribunal with me the doctors asked me what happened to me in Leicester I told them I walked the yellow lines all day and all night, I told them that I was going to be the king of Scotland all I can remember after that they had put me on a section three which could last up to six months unless you got better and won your tribunal. The doctor started me on some new medication he said it was an eighteen-week course and that I would have to have my blood pressure taken and blood taken every week my new medication was called clozaril. My appointment had come through to go back down to Glenfied hospital for a ct scan from when I had my seizure on Ashby ward after my scan the nurses took me back I had to wait to get my results back, after a few weeks on the ward I started to get audited from the antipsychrcotric drugs my skin was crawling my feet were shuffling this was making me higher, on the ward I could not sit still I would run up and down the corridors dead fast leistering to my music and singing a long, in ward round I asked the doctor what he was treating me for and he said schizophrenia and I said what when I am as high as a kite , I had my first breakdown when I was thirty three and a man could have schizophrenia from sixteen to the age of twenty two, I am now thirty eight you are getting this all wrong and I stormed out of ward round I did not like this one bit then a seen a nurse and told him to pull the trigger six nurses crab hold of me and took me to seclusion they took my cloths off and my Jew rely  then left me and locked the door, I felt like history was repeating its self what had happened to me in 1995 I got a lot of anger out I was in and out of seclusion most of the week until I got the anger out of my system . I still continue to be high I can not tell you what happened every day as I was to ill to remember most of it even when Janet came to visit me I did not really know she was here most of the time. There was a German patient in here I can remember talking to him I asked him if he lived in Germany he said yes but he could not speak much English I asked one of the nurses why he was here they said a couple of years ago he was on holiday in England and while on holiday he became un well so he was taken to Belvoir unit for treatment, so this time when he became ill he got a one way ticket to England and made his way back here for treatment. Always at six in the morning he would get up to watch the news and one morning I put a bed sheet over my head I went up to him and scared him, I was always getting up to mischief one night I took a bed from another patient room and put it my room it was really funny when he went to tell the nurses he had no bed in his room, then I would go in the other patients rooms and hide there cloths the nurses were looking for cloths every where, the nurse said this is not funny he seemed like a proper warden to me. I was still on the same medication even though it did not seem to be working for me I seemed to be getting worse instead of better, they still checked my blood pressure and took my blood every week they weighed me I was thirteen stone when I went over there now I was 11 and half stone and eating well but I was on the go all the time still not sleeping at night I was running up and down the ward with a sheet over my head pretending to be a ghost and when day time came I was still on the go I could not settle or sit down, at night time  when I was in my room the nurse would look through the peep hole to see what I was doing I would be laying under the bed lifting it and down doing press ups. I got my results back from the hospital they said I had Neurleptic Malignant Syndrome caused by adverse reaction to antipsychiotic drugs.

Christmas day Janet came to visit me, the nurses watched me whilst I opened my presents then they let us have some time together in the small television room. When Janet left I went into seclusion and listened to my music tears running down my face.

The week after Christmas was New Years Eve I asked the nurses if Janet was going to come and see they and me told me that she wasn't because there was no buses that ran on New Years Eve. I thought to myself Oh Fuck what the hell am I going to do in here? I'm a Scotchman I told the nurses to pull the trigger and they said are you sure and I replied yes! Six or seven nurse grabbed hold of me and took me into seclusion and pinned me face down to the floor. I was in so much rage and anger I told the nurses that I was not there to hurt them. I almost stood all the way back up I was that strong they told me to lie back down and that they have to give me a small injection to calm me down. I said to them that I wasn't taking any more bad shit; the doctors can stick it up their arse. I told them that I was staying in seclusion for three days and I wasn't coming back out.

In seclusion all I did was walk around I didn't sleep at all, the next morning they came and opened the door and the nurse saw that I had calmed down a lot they told me that I could go back into my bedroom but I said no I wanted to stay in seclusion for one more night. So they gave me some breakfast, it seemed a long while being in seclusion for two days and nights but it was quiet and the air was cool not like the seclusion on Ashby ward. The next day the nurses coached me to come out and to go into my bedroom which that night I had a good nights sleep for the first time since October my body and brain started to shut down. The doctor came back from his Christmas break, I went into ward round and he was disbelieving that he saw a different man in me. I told him that I was not taking any more bad shit and any more anti psychiatric. So I asked him if I could have some Carbamazepine slow release and he said yes. I was so relieved that a weight had been pulled off my shoulders and a felt as though I could have kisses him. I left ward round thinking look what you can do when you put your foot down. I had been asking for Carbamazepine for five years now on and off now I have finally got my voice was herd, he started me off with four hundred milligrams then I went up to six hundred milligrams daily. I knew it would take me a couple of months to get well what I'd been through.

I had my manager's tribunal coming up soon to look forward to. First thing I did was ring Janet up to tell her the good news and she told me that I sounded better like I was a different person. I told her that things were looking up for me now and it wouldn't be long before I was getting out of here and back onto Ashby ward. I told Janet I loved her then I put the phone down. All I had to do now on the ward was relax and rest the nurses saw a big difference in me.

On the twentieth of January I was watching the snooker master final in the small television room. Steven Henry was playing Mark Williams a patient walked in a sat down it got to the black ball and the patient turned the channel over. At that time I was really pissed off and I said to him what the fuck did you do that for I was watching that and threw some water over him. He stood straight up and started punching me in the face he hit me twenty to twenty five times, his last few punches wouldn't have hurt a fly I said is that the hardest you can hit mate first, a nurse could see me from a distance and what was going on, they came over to me and the patient that hit me was in disbelief because I was still standing and didn't flinch. The nurse took me into the medication room I had a bust nose and two black eyes. They gave me some Paracetamol and cleaned my nose up. I told the nurse that they better put him in seclusion and they told me that they had. I couldn't see what he had done to me because there were no mirrors on the ward.

My manager's tribunal came through we have a meeting over at Bradgate unit with my solicitor and Janet came as well with my doctor from Ashby ward. They asked me at the meeting that my diagnoses were and my doctor said Schizo effective Disorder. One of the judges off the panel said that he had never herd of it they asked me if my medication was working and the doctor said it appeared to be. They asked me if my seizure was life threatening and the doctor said yes. Me Janet and the ward manager from Belvoir ward left the room not long after the hospital managers came to see us and what a great support Janet had given me. That they had never seen anything like this before. They said we are not able to lift your section but we can give you 17 order which allows patients to leave the ward for six hours a day, then return back onto the ward. I asked them if I could stay in Belvoir ward so that I could feel better about my doctor before I went back to Ashby ward. The doctor wanted to see me in ward round he asked me why I didn't hit the other patient back. I told him at the time it felt like it was a set up and if I had hit him back I would have lost me Carbamazepine. They just looked at me and said nothing I told them if he comes after me again I would give him a hard time. I knew it was going to take me a couple of weeks to forgive him. When we went in for dinner I would sit next to him he would only eat his pudding and then run off. All I wanted to do was to scare him off this went on for week then I shook his hand and he went back onto his own ward.

My Carbamazepine started to kick in I was listening to my music but I wasn't singing any more. I rang and asked Janet if she would get me some CD's. My first CD was my ero 1985 The Pleasure Dome bye Holly Johnson, my second one was Only The Strong Survive by Billy Paul and the third was 1988 when my daughter was born. Fleetwood Mac and also Boy zone. When I first met Janet I looked at these as my personal CD's, this music and Janet would pull me out of hospital, I knew it would take Janet a couple of weeks to get some of these CD's but I could listen to them when I got back onto Ashby ward. I just kept myself to myself on the ward I would talk to the nurses I talked to the German patient and Id play pool with the nurses but then they stopped playing with me because I kept winning. Which I felt they didn't like loosing to somebody who is mad.

My sleep started to get better they gave me Zopilone and six hundred milligrams of Carbamazepine. I had escorted walks around the grounds and not long after I could go out on my own. I asked the nurses why am I allowed to go on my own when we are on a locked ward and they said because we know you will come back. Then shortly after that the doctor let me have leave on the Fourteenth of February for six hours. It was great to go back to my flat even though it was only for a few hours and the time went quick. On the next ward round the doctor asked me how my leave went and I said great and I asked him if I could go back onto Ashby ward? He asked me how I felt about my doctor? I said ok now so later on that afternoon they took me back to Ashby ward, the feeling was great to get back onto my own ward. I could have all my toiletries and my mobile phone in my own room so that I could ring Janet and have private conversations. I went into the day room and made myself a drink and then went into the smoke room. Some of the patients asked me what it was like on a locked ward I told them that it was hard work and that they wouldn't like it over there. They asked me how long I had spent over there and I said twenty-two weeks and by now it was the end of February 2000.

Wednesday was ward round I went into see the doctor I told him that I had taken a good beating over there. I told him that I wanted him to know that I was only a danger to myself and that the only person I had ever put in an ambulance was myself. He said that he wanted to make me better and gave me some Lamotrigine fifty milligrams but I would have to take it slowly in case of any side effects. I felt that he really wanted to help me and I ended up loving my enemy then I left ward round.

Janet came to visit me every other day for six hours, which kept me strong on the ward. The doctor started to give me more leave, as he was pleased with my progress.

The Lamotrigine and the Carbamazepine worked well together. I was in more control of my life and my illness. My favourite music that Janet had brought for me was the pleasure dome the power of love, I would listen to it for a long while before I went to bed. The next day I went into seclusion to sing this because it was a good room to sing in. The doctor came onto the ward and didn't like it because I was in seclusion singing loudly. I came out of seclusion and talked to the doctor he asked me what I was listening to so I gave him my CD player to listen to my music. I told the doctor that I wanted to sing in seclusion to get it out of my system, he told me not to do it again.

Then I started to get more and more leave the nurses could see how well I was doing so they let me have over night stays. I was handling my leave very well but when I went back onto the ward my mood would change again because I didn't want to be here anymore. The doctor gave me a week's leave and told me to come back for ward round and he discharged me on the 29<sup>th</sup> of March 2000.

CHAPTER NINE.

Fresh Start (April 1<sup>st</sup> 2001).

Nice to have a good night sleep in my own bed. Later that week I opened my mail, I had to go thought it all over again that my rent hadn't been paid whilst I was n hospital. The council sent me a letter telling me that they had stopped paying my rent because my benefits had changed to a lower income with me being in hospital. They said that I wasn't entitled to my rent benefit. The landlord had also sent me a letter for one thousand pound rent arrears; this stress was enough to put me back into hospital. I thought I would end up losing my flat, I thought no way would the landlord let me off this time. I told the council and my landlord that I would contact my local MP. I made an appointment he looked into the matter for me, when he got back to me he said he was sorry there was nothing that he could do to help me. The law had been going for fifty years and that it could not be changed I felt gutted and so guilty inside. You wouldn't find many landlords like I had. My landlord was upset and he said to my MP this is the second time this is happened I was feeling so much stress at the time I had a lot on my mind. My CPN wrote to my landlord explaining everything, my landlord came to see me he told me that it wasn't my fault, that it was the system and he let me off with the rent arrears. I felt that this law should be changed, there is so many people that it can effect and they cannot do anything about it.

My friends stopped ringing me Janet would come and see me in the morning before she started work. I was finding it hard going into the shops to do my shopping sometimes I would just walk out if there were to many people in there, then go back later when it wasn't so busy. When I got my concentration back along with my confidence. Janet and I continued to see each other; we would go out for a drink at the weekend. Being in hospital for so long had made me lose the taste for drink whereas a few years ago I used to drink a lot. Now I was lucky if I could drink three pints and most of the time I didn't enjoy it.

A couple of months went by I contacted the Salvation Army to search for my father I told them as much information as I could, that he had two brothers that still lived in Scotland and that I thought that he was living in London. It took them a while for them to get back to me they told me that he was not living in London and that he hadn't remarried and that they couldn't really find any more information out about him for me. I still continued to do my befriending scheme as I was feeling better at the time, I would take one of the befriended out for a game of pool and sometimes if he didn't feel like it we would stop in and have a chat. Listening to all the people's problems would take my mind off of my own, I enjoyed helping other people.

I needed a holiday after what I had been through so I booked a week in Greece for me and Janet being out of the country made me feel like a different person it was just what I needed, It made me feel better about myself. Life seemed to be getting better for me; I got a car in October, which seemed to help me get about a lot. Living on my own seemed to be getting me down and my flat was only small and very cold in the winter. Janet and I seemed to be getting on well, as we had been together for nearly two years so Janet asked me if I wanted to move in with her. This was near Christmas time. After the New Year we felt that we needed a fresh start and a different house Janet's house was damp and needed a lot of work doing to it. The council said that they couldn't do the work whilst we were living in it. At the end of January they offered us a house in Coalville but it wouldn't be ready for a couple of months. My CPN told me I must be mad taking it on because of the condition it was in and he told me to be careful incase it made me ill again. When we got the keys to the house it wasn't liveable it had to be decorated from top to bottom. Janet's family helped us a lot with the decorating; I enjoyed doing the work it would keep my mind on the job and not thinking about other things. Some of the jobs I had never done before. The garden was the biggest job it was one hundred and fifty feet long. I was working that hard I wasn't sleeping properly everything had to be done as quickly as possible. After we had got the house straight and most of the garden we decided to get married in Scotland In May the following year. My fortieth birthday was coming up so we had a small party with family and friends at the house. Having things to do made me feel really well and getting a fresh start in life was going well for a change. I stopped doing the befriending scheme as I felt that I needed a change as I had been doing it for seven years. In June 2004 I started as a volunteer with the peoples forum. This is a group ran by and for service users in the county of Leicestershire and Rutland. We have all personal experiences of mental distress. Some of the work that we do involves taking service users views to the healthcare providers.

CHAPTER TEN.


Playing snooker in the premier league.

It seemed to be going well it was April 2003, me and Janet went to the Crucible Theatre in Sheffield to watch Ronnie O'Sullivan against Marco Fu in the first round match. Ronnie knocked in a 147 break it was a great night for me to see a 147 to go in live. On the way back home I said to Janet I am going to start the game back up as a hobby now that the house was finished.

A week later I walked into my local snooker hall potters and made myself a member. I hadn't played snooker for over ten years. I used to play a little bit before my first breakdown; I didn't want anybody to know about me having a illness. I started playing the young lads at first I wasn't playing very well. I looked on the Internet for a BBC coach. Who I then contacted the closest to me was Nottingham I went there every week on a Monday morning he improved my game onto another level. I was knocking forty breaks in after a month's time I started playing in the Sunday knockouts at Potters. I lost my first match because I was nervous. The month after I got to the semi-finals. I signed up for the first division to play for the team every Monday night, playing around the Leicester area there were four players in the team and you would only play two frames. I'd mostly play away so the young lads could play when we was at home, I would win most of my matches away and draw some. I still continued to see my coach in Nottingham. I knocked my first fifty breaks in, in October playing against a friend. My highest break in a match was thirty-three but I was a good safety player. I continued playing in the monthly knock outs and get to the semi-finals. My handicap when I first started was seventy-seven and my lowest handicap went down to thirty five they worked it out on black ball. Every time I got to the semi-final I would loose seven points. Years 2004 October I knocked in my first hundred and two break whilst playing a friend.

I fount out that Jimmy White was playing Alex Higgins in an exhibition match at the Barbican Centre in York. I went with a friend we got tickets for the VIP lounge so we could meet the players and get a signed autograph on photos. Jimmy White has been my idol since the late eighties and I first saw him playing at the crucible in 1991 against Stephen Hendry. I signed up for the premier league it was still playing around Leicester but there were eight teams I can remember playing at the 147 club the closest I got was down to the colours and I ended up loosing. Most of my games went down to the colours but I lost my bottle and never really seemed to have it takes to play snooker at a higher level. When it came down to it I just couldn't do it there was so much expectation I didn't want to let the other team members down. All through the season I never won a game I would loose sleep the night before I was due to play. I can remember going to see my coach crying on the way I would dry my tears then go into the snooker hall. I'd pot some blacks then I would start laughing I new I was heading for a breakdown.

It was getting near to Christmas and I knew I wasn't very well so when the Cpn came to visit me I told her how I was feeling and that I didn't want to go in hospital over Christmas. So she went and had a word with the doctor when she came back she said the doctor wants you to up your medication Carbamazepine to 800mg and he gave me some diazepam 5mg to take no more than 30mg a day. This was the maximum dose to shut me down. I knew myself it was too late to nip it in the bud this time I was drugged up to the eye balls, my life was all out of control I knew after the new year that I would have to hand myself in this went on until February. On the 8th February 2005 the CPN came to my house I would hide myself away from Janet and the family down the garden shed the CPN saw me down the shed and she said that she was concerned about me and would I go with her to the hospital and I said yes!

## CHAPTER ELEVEN

My Fourth Nervous Breakdown.

February the 8th 2005 I went upstairs and packed a bag, I came back down stairs and asked Janet to let me settle for a week before she came to visit me. We both had a cry and a cuddle then I got in the CPN's car. I knew where I was going to end up. My thoughts were that I would only be in hospital for four weeks. I thought to myself my brains been through a bit of a battering and that I had done well to stay out of hospital for five years. I had a chat with the CPN on the way and told her that I had to get my sleep right. I made my way onto Ashby ward at the Bradgate unit, the CPN told me to go and sit down whilst they sorted me a room out. I had to go through the normal procedure of then checking my bag. The nurses were nice and friendly to me. Nothing had seemed to change much since last time that I was on the ward. I knew it was going to be hard to get used to the surroundings again. The nurses knew me from last time so they gave me my own room because they knew that I couldn't settle in a dormitory. That night I didn't sleep much I was all over the place in and out of the smoke room.

Ward round was Wednesday morning at ten thirty I had to go in and see the doctor. There were between sixteen and eighteen people it hit me like a tonne of bricks. I felt like there were extra people in there just because I was there.

# I THOUGHT I WAS THE KING OF SCOTLAND

The doctor asked me what had happened to me I told him that me and Janet went on holiday last year and the car had broken down and if it hadn't off been for my plastic friend which was my credit card I would have had to travel back on the train. We were without the car for three days and the bill came to over five hundred pounds. The next day we had to leave the cottage I said to Janet lets go down to Newquay. We pulled up at the harbour car park I told my doctor I could remember when I was seventeen I first went water skiing there and I looked up at the hotel and I said I would love to take a women there one day. I said to Janet lets go and book in for the night this made me feel so happy stopping there for the night because of the car breaking down. We had a good walk around the shops I was telling them that Janet was one in a million, I was all out of control I didn't think that I had done myself any favours telling them all that and talking fast as well. I didn't mention anything about my snooker but I knew it had section two written all over it not much happened on the ward after that apart from I started to settle down and my sleep started to get better. I was getting four hours sleep I phoned Janet and asked her to come and see me a week later I asked her if she would visit me every other day. She would come on the ward at twelve o'clock and bring some lunch with her we would go off the ward and have something to eat.

I started smoking cigars again. I told Janet that they had put me on some new medication Risperidone three milligrams they kept me on my current medication I didn't know how it was going

Jimmy Gilmour

to suit me. The days Janet didn't come to visit me I was unsettled I would go to my room a lot and just lay there for hours then I would force myself to go into the smoke room and have a coffee and a cigar and talk to the other patients.

A few weeks later being on Risperidone I started to get very paranoid and talk to God after my medication at night time, then I would listen to my music sometimes I would sing and sometime I wouldn't. I was asking god if I had ever been here before in a previous life I back to the same old bazaar behaviour as before. I would get a sense of feeling that I was in Scotland in Clayne Castle, thinking I was going back there with my ancestors I thought that I was a Viking and I would travel from Scotland to Greece. The reason why I had to write this book was to find out where the king of Scotland really came from? I was having false beliefs again I can remember talking to my mother after my first breakdown I asked her why did she leave Scotland and come to live in England? She said that she had hired a private detective and found out that my father was having an affair. I got it into my head that she was Greek and that my mother wasn't my mother and my father went to Greece to fetch me and fly me back to Scotland then brought me back to England and that I had to do ten years in and out of a psychiatric hospital and walk all day and all night all around Leicester following the yellow lines. That I would have to find my Father and he would show me the way how to be the king of Scotland but I would keep asking God if my father was alive but my mother told me that he had two brothers that lived in Scotland and that they may be able to help me find him.

The night staff would listen outside my door that I was talking to myself. The duty doctor came to see me the next morning and he asked me if I was hearing voices this went on for a week the duty doctor would come into my room and I kept telling them that I had never heard voices that I was having a conversation with god. I did tell my regular doctor in ward round were the king of Scotland came from he said you must have had a passport when you was younger and I said I don't know about that. I told him that the Risperidone wasn't doing me any good and he didn't answer me. I can remember eating my breakfast and a new patient was on the ward I nicknamed him Blondie he said I'm here to hit you I didn't think much of it at the time because he wasn't very well and hadn't been on the ward long. I kept my distance from him I did learn through the years of being in hospital when some body comes in fresh that I didn't want to get beat up again every time I saw him he was eye balling me I thought oh fuck! I was getting anxiety attacks hiding myself in my room didn't want to go into the smoke room and have a confrontation with him. I started getting angry with myself my muscles were tightening up racing thoughts going through my head really fast. I was getting scared what the fuck is happening to me this was total bazaar behaviour I packed my bag walked straight into the smoke room and hit Blondie once it all happened so fast one of the nurses came straight over to me and put me into seclusion I still had my watch and my jewellery on

I knew that I would get punished for what I had just done. I was calm in seclusion my feet were suffering and could not stop still and I was suffering from dystonic extra pyramidal side effects. Stiffness and trembling. I was getting up and down of the mattress walking from corner to corner I never lay down once they kept me in there for twenty three hours. They opened the door to give me something to eat. I didn't eat a thing all the nurses came in later with the doctor. He said you are going to Belvoir ward they told me that I would have to wait for a bit longer until they got my a bed over there. Eight nurses took me over I felt like they were marching me to prison I didn't like it one bit having to go there again. Looking back I wish that I had asked the nurses for two blueys. If I had taken the blue tablets they would have calmed me down and I would not have hit Blondie because I have always been a man that would walk away from trouble. But I clearly wasn't very well at the time the atmosphere on the ward was very tense not long after on the ward the nurse was reading his paper and I slapped his paper they grabbed holt of me and put me straight into seclusion they took all my clothes off apart from my underwear they striped off all my dignity they gave me a blue top and blue bottoms, I felt like a Muppet. A few hours later they let me out they said that I would have to stop in the seclusion area all night. I had to see the doctor the next day and he wanted to know why I had done it, I told him that I was all out of control and my medication wasn't suiting me I couldn't believe what he had done he upped my medication from three mg of

Risperidone to four mg daily a few day later I began to have seizures again the nurses put me in seclusion so no one else could see what was happening to me there was no way the doctor had read my medical notes from last time.

The nurses knew straight away that Neurleptic malignant syndrome had come back again they told me that the doctor didn't realise and that they had put my medication back down to two mg daily I wasn't well enough to argue with them and tell them that I didn't want to take the medication but the seizures wasn't as bad this time. A few days later my social worker came to see me she gave me a piece of paper and told me as from now I was on a section three I spent a month on Belvoir ward then I went back over to Ashby ward.

I was relieved that I was getting out of Belvoir ward. There were a couple of items of mine that went missing, one was my gold chain that my wife had brought me and I would not be able to replace it. The other was my bible (The first testament), which a patient gave me before I went onto belvoir ward. I was looking forward to reading the bible because I had never read it before. Ten o'clock that night I went for my medication, I refused the three milligrams of Risperidone. I told the nurse I only wanted two milligrams of it because I could be at risk of having another seizure. He said you would have to sort it out with the doctor in ward round.

It was nice to use my mobile phone that night to ring Janet up because you weren't allowed to use them on Belviour ward. I was due to see the doctor in ward round he told me that I had to carry on taking three milligrams of Risperidone. I told that it was too much of a cocktail that I was taking six hundred milligrams of Carbamazepine, one hundred milligrams of Lamotrigine and five milligrams of Diazepam. I explained to him the Risperidone can suit some people but it doesn't suit me, I stormed out of ward round. A few weeks past and I was due to see my daughter it was her birthday and we had a nice chat. Not long after the weather started to pick up I was allowed off the ward to go into the day centre to play pool with some of the other patients. I would spend two hours of the ward. Snooker was on the television and I started to relax I realised that I had to stay on the three milligrams of Risperidone or the doctor would hold me until the end of my section. I wasn't happy about it as I was suffering from side effects soar shoulders and a soar back.

The managers meeting was coming up they said that they wouldn't be able to lift my section but they would try and get me some more leave I did well in the meeting, my regular doctor wasn't there it was the duty doctor. After the meeting I had to go and see my own doctor on Ashby ward. I was in there for a long time; I told him that I was having contact with god. I felt like he was trying to trick me I asked him if I could have one or two nights leave and he said im sorry what you just told me, I am concerned about you so leave will not be possible. Maybe next week.

Two new CPN's came on the ward they told us they were from County Outreach and when I got my section lifted I would be in there care and have a different doctor. I said oh great that would be a positive thing as I have lost my faith in my regular doctor. They explained things would be done differently. That I would have better care out in the community, everything would be done at home, no outpatients visits to the doctor or CPA meeting they would come to your house and see you with your doctor and when it was your cpa review they would do that at home as well. Their job is to keep you out of hospital as best as they can, even if they have to visit your home more that once a day. The next ward round I told the doctor about me changing over to a new team he said that sounds good for you. I told him that when I get out of hospital I would like to go to Scotland for a few days after what I had been through. He said I will let you go home for a week then come back and see me. It was nice to get back home I knew when I got discharged that I would come off the Risperidone but I would tell my new CPN. The week went by fast it was time to go back and see the doctor he asked me what I had been doing, painting some fence panels and watching the television. He asked if I went out anywhere and I said no. I said I would like you to discharge me now doctor so I can go and have my holiday! When was you thinking of going? Monday to Friday, he said you can go but I wont lift your section I said that I wasn't happy about what he had said. I said that I wasn't travelling all that way with a section hanging over me I wouldn't be able to enjoy myself.

After further talks with the doctor he said go home for another week then come back and see and me and I will think about lifting your section. I relaxed back at home I couldn't wait to get back and see the doctor. When I went to see the doctor I told him that everything had gone well at home and he said that I was well and he was going to lift my section. My new CPN was in ward round as well I was under the doctors care for seven years and we shock hands and he wished me all the best I was in hospital for four months!

CHAPTER TWELVE

News of my dad

The second week in June 2005, it was a Monday and Janet and I went to Scotland for a short break. Which I had booked a guesthouse on the Internet; we woke up early and set off on our journey. We stopped off a Gretna Green and had something to eat and a walk around the outlet village. It brought back lovely memories as we married there in 2002. We travelled further into Ayr; the guesthouse wasn't far from the sea front. The landlady was nice and friendly she told us where could get a nice meal, in a pub just around the corner. It used to be a church before the brewery brought it. The next day we went sight seeing the weather was really nice and the last time the weather was that hot was in 1976. a couple of days later at breakfast we were talking to the landlady I told her that I was born in Scotland and I had moved to England with my parents went I was two years old. After a few years my parents separated and I lost contact with my father. I was telling the landlady how I tried to find my father but over the years I couldn't find any more information about him. She asked me what part of Scotland he was from I said Catherine. And that he had two brothers she said that that wasn't far from Ayr. She said leave it with me and later she would look it up on the Internet. To see if there was anybody with that name living in the area.

The next day when we were leaving to go home she gave us a name and address and a telephone number. I wanted to go to the address but Janet said no wait until we get back home. We made our way safely back home. I thought that I had done really well after being in hospital for four months. We didn't know what to do whether to contact them or not, so a few days later Janet rang up and explained who we were. They told us yes it was my father's brother but they were sorry that my father had passed away in 1985 in London. Janet came downstairs and told me the news, all I could think about at that time was I would have only been twenty-four years old when he died. I've been wondering all these years if I would be able to find him and have a father son relationship with him.

I thought to myself I am going to stay strong for this would the news give me another breakdown? With me only just coming out of hospital. I had to have extra CPN visits twice a week. I wanted to go to London to pay my respects and find which crematorium his ashes were buried, a couple of weeks later Janet and I was going to go but a terrorist attack broke out, so we decided not to go.

A few months later I started to take ill I wasn't getting much sleep I was coming downstairs in the middle of the night and eating. These were early warning signs for me. I was getting paranoid and also suffering from the highs and lows. The CPN came to see me and I lied to them about how ill I really was if your not honest with them and tell them how your really feeling, how can they help you? I started with bazaar behaviour taking things down the shed wearing two to three layers of clothing, not speaking to Janet or wanting to be in the same room as her. My life was all out of control and I was giving Janet a hard time. I kept disappearing and wouldn't tell her where I was going or what I was doing. We had a bit of money in the bank that I drew out without Janet knowing, my daughter was stopping over the that night when she went to bed I told Janet that I needed a break and when my daughter had gone to college the next morning, I was going away for a couple of days.

## CHAPTER THIRTEEN

Scotland on my own

Wednesday morning, November 3$^{rd}$ 2005. I packed my bag and took my snooker cue and went away for a short break to sort my head out. Janet said look after yourself, I didn't tell her where I was going. I had made my mind up where I was going; I made my way up to the M1 and stopped at Gretna Green for a break. I got back into my car and ended up at Preswick airport I parked on the long stay car park, I had my passport with me and went to see if there were any flights to Greece or Spain. There wasn't any going that day; I asked one of the ladies if I could have a refund. I rang Janet up and told her where I was and where I wanted to go. She said your not going anywhere like that. Thinking about it later I was glad that I didn't leave the country, with me not being very well. I found the nearest hotel and tried to get some sleep but didn't get much sleep that night. After breakfast I rang my uncle up and told him that I was in Scotland and asked him if I could come and visit him. And he said yes, I went and had a shower and got myself ready I arrived at my uncle's house he knew that I was behaving strangely. He made me a cup of tea we talked a bit about my father. I wasn't taking a lot in at the time. I told him a bit about myself that I was married and had a daughter and that I like playing snooker. I went to my car and got my snooker cue out I asked him if he would look after it for me, he told me that Stephen Hendry didn't live far from him. I said he is the king of snooker. I was waiting for my uncle to tell me how I could be the king of Scotland. I knew then I was never going to come true. I gave him my mobile number and a photo of Janet and my daughter. He spoke to me a bit about his grandchildren. I gave him some money and asked him if he would save it for me, I was begging to feel high again at this time, so a told him I was leaving. He asked me where I was going I said into Ayr I shook his hand gave him a kiss and said goodbye.

I parked on a small car park in Ayr and went to look around some shops, I was looking for satellite navigation with me being so high my concentration wasn't very good, I was loosing all sense of direction I thought that I would never find my way back home. I was getting frightened and scared. A map wouldn't have been much use, as I wouldn't of bin able to read it. I was walking around the town centre in circles; I was going through so much mental pain my brain was in turmoil by that time. I had forgotten where I had parked me car and only had half an hour left on the parking ticket. I was having visions that my car would be towed away I was going to ring my uncle and tell him that I had lost my car but I knew that he wouldn't be able to help me. I saw a taxi and asked the driver if he could help me I told the driver I couldn't remember where I parked my car and could he help me find it? It was a small car park in the town centre next to a pub. We drove around a few places I started to panic. Then he found it for me gave him ten pound and told him to keep the change. My brain had gone back to a few months ago when Janet and I had stayed in the guesthouse I was looking for my hotel but couldn't find it. I stopped and asked someone if he knew where it was it said Preswick hotel on my keying. He said try the local police station mate. I thought he was taking the piss. I came back to my senses and I realised my hotel was in Preswick not Ayr. I went back to my hotel and told the manager that I was leaving and could I have my bill? I travelled back into Ayr it was just starting to get dark. I parked up at the sea front and went for a long walk trying to clear my head ready for the journey back home. Later I filled up with petrol and made my way to Gretna Green. I stopped there and had something to eat.

Then made my way to Scotch corner roundabout. I took the wrong turning I don't know how it happened but I ended up in Cumbria by this time it was ten o'clock at night I parked up and had something to eat and a rest. I rang Janet up and told her where I was and that I was stopping the night and would be back tomorrow afternoon I still felt on a bit of a high so instead of stopping the night I decided to come back home. Thinking I could drive anywhere and not get tired after driving for a couple of hours I did eventually find the M6. This was scary but the some of the sights I had seen were breath taking. I knew if I stopped on the M6 I would soon see a sign saying Leicester I drove a bit further that I realised I had missed the junction that I wanted. I was only sixteen miles away from Blackpool I pulled over at the nearest café and had a drink, then I spoke to a gentlemen and told him that I was lost and wanted to get to Leicester could he give me some directions for the nearest toll bridge? He said you have gone a bit further up and he gave me the directions. I got back into my car I was enjoying the driving as the music made me high. I was so relived that I was heading in the right direction. I made my way back home it was early hours of Saturday morning I just had enough petrol to get home I drove over a thousand miles in three days and I knew I was heading for another breakdown. After I had been back home a few hours I told Janet to ring the CPN's and tell them that I needed to go into hospital for a couple of weeks.

## CHAPTER FOURTEEN

Back in Hospital

November 5th 2005, at ten am two CPN's came to my house I did not hesitate. I told them that I needed to go back into hospital. Janet had my bag packed ready. It seemed like a long drive there, I thought that the Brandon unit was at the back of the Bradgate unit my old ward. The CPN's told me that we were going to the general hospital. I had to walk up three flights of stairs. There was a locked door, a small corridor with some rooms either side. There was a small area with a desk and above it said Herrick ward. The nurse's office was to the left and the treatment room was to the right. There was a small smoke room, which was very dirty and smoked up.

The women sleeping quarter was to the left and the men's were to the right. There was a nice little quiet room there, which had just been freshly decorated. They only had to small room plus the dormitory. One of the small rooms was next door to the kitchen. They had a small living room area where you would eat and watch the television. There wasn't much space to walk around I knew that I wasn't going to get used to these surroundings. It was not fit for a psychiatric hospital I knew I was going to miss my old ward straight away as you could just walk outside the smoke room and get some fresh air. I was still feeling a bit high I never really knew where I was, they put me in a dormitory that night and told me that I would have to sleep there until they could get me a single room. They gave me Zopiclone I didn't sleep that much that night I was lucky if I got two hours. I always showered and shaved in hospital every morning no matter how bad I was feeling inside. I had some breakfast the nurse's felt so close to you, everything felt tight they would sit next to you and watch you eat I felt so uncomfortable, you wouldn't get that in prison.

I didn't bother ringing Janet for a couple of days I rang my mum instead and told her that my dad died and I had met my uncle in Scotland and that I wanted the doctors to transfer me to a Scottish psychiatric hospital. I told her how much I loved her she asked me where I was I said that I didn't know and that the building was three stories high. That they had put me somewhere different. Mum was very quiet so I said goodbye. Later I had to see that doctor I was nervous as hell, I had one sit each side of me I told them that I was under a lot of stress and that I had lost a lot of sleep and the news about my father made me all out of control and I feel that my life had been turned up side down. Two breakdowns in one year, one doctor said it sounds like your bi-polar has come back. I thought to my self thank god for they have got my illness right. He said that we will keep you on your current medication and keep taking you sleeping pills. I thought that he was a nice doctor because he didn't section me and that would be a good thing for my marriage and myself. I left ward round and I said to myself I've just got to grin and bare it. I couldn't have any escorted walks until next week they gave me my own bedroom, my only problem in here would be fresh air. I started smoking cigars in the smoke room, I still had thoughts in my head about being the king of Scotland this time I knew I couldn't tell any body about it, then I went into the quiet room and a doctor asked if he could chat with me. He asked me if I had secret powers I said yes but I didn't want to talk about it anymore. Next time I seen my psychiatrist I asked him if I could have some fresh air and that it was important to me and could he get me transferred to a Scottish hospital. He said I don't think Scottish laws will work like that, wait until you are feeling a bit better, he said you need some Olanzapine. We will start you on five mg; you will need this tablet to keep you out of hospital. I believed him.

It was nice to get out and have some fresh air; it felt fantastic because I am a fresh air person. I had a chat with the nurse whilst we were walking around I told him that I was worried about the stigma and I felt that I would never be able to play snooker again. The pupils at school should learn about mental health problems in the school curriculum, sociology.

People found out in the snooker hall about my bi-polar disorder this was also another part of my breakdown I had been in hospital for two weeks. My sleep was getting better they upped my Olanzapine to ten mg daily. This knocked me out for six, I would eat during the night and I was doing so well. A couple of days later I felt as if I was going to blow I asked the nurses to give me two blueys which are Lorazepan. they put me in seclusion where I got rid of some anger. They let me out after three hours; I wasn't looking forward to ward round. The doctor said my medication wasn't working and that he was going to put me on Lithium next week. I couldn't be bothered to tell him that I was struggling for fresh air and that my Olanzapine was too higher of a dose. I thought to myself why put me on Lithium a week later why not now? Does he want to keep me in here longer? The doctor asked me if he could see my wife and I said yes. I rang Janet up later and asked her to come and visit me. I said im not going to get any better now in this shit hole! I rang my daughter and asked if she would come and visit me as well. I started to come back to my senses knowing that you can't run away from the stigma. That I had a wife that loved me. Janet visited and so did my daughter. Janet was in with the doctor for a long while then I had to see the doctor after. They started me on Lithium and cut me back down to five mg of Olanzapine a week later I discharged myself on the fourth of December. A year later Herrick ward closed.

Being Determined

Fifth of December 2005, it was nice to get back home and get back into my own bed. I was going to give Lithium a try for three to six months. The New Year past but my mood was still low, I realised Lithium wasn't working for me. In March I went to see my uncle in Scotland to go and get my snooker cue back. They let me stay over night. We had a good chat and everything seemed different. They knew I was acting strange last time when I visited them. I told my uncle about my illness, that I have bi-polar disorder and that I was taking medication for it. I left the next morning to go back home, after I got back home I decided to ask the doctor to come and visit me, as I couldn't get my mood right. I needed to be on an even keel and the Lithium wasn't doing that for me. I told the doctor that I had given Lithium a go but it wasn't working for me I couldn't get my mood right and asked if I could go back onto my old medication. Carbamazepine four hundred milligrams daily and Lamotrigine hundred and fifty milligrams twice a day. The doctor said you would need to take two-point five mg of Olanzapine.

It took me until July 2006 to get well I was so glad that I had got my old medication back I felt like that it had really fucked my life up for over six months. If your not happy with the medication you must tell you doctor. Nothing much happened after that apart from January 2007 I started to play snooker with my CPN in my local snooker hall. I hit a mini crisis in May the weather wasn't very good, it rained a lot, I didn't sleep very good I got high as a kite. I went to the golf range and played golf something, which I hadn't done in over thirteen years. Then I drove to Leicester and went bowling, I was hitting a strike nearly every time. Sweat was pouring off me. I came back home I knew I was acting strange the CPN's came around to visit me I told them that they better get the doctor around as soon as possible. Something just dawned on me about my medication that I needed six hundred milligrams of Carbamazepine not four hundred. I upped my medication myself before the doctor came. I knew I needed some thing else to keep me out of hospital so the doctor told me to take five milligrams of Olanzapine and he also gave me two milligrams of Lorazepan to shut me down. This worked it did the trick and kept me out of hospital.

After two weeks I started to come of Lorazepan by taking one milligram then half. By August I started to get my life back in control a couple of months passed I was still doing voluntary work for people forum and I volunteered for the ward forums, to go back on my old ward at the Bradgate unit. It took twelve weeks to process for Leicestershire partner trust, so now I go on the wards every two weeks and listen and try and help the other service users. Then I put in for peer advocacy work for Lamp as a volunteer, I got an interview in November and got the place January 2008, I started my seven-week training course. On the twenty eighth of February I got my certificate of achievement for successfully completing the peer advocacy training course my life couldn't get any better I feel like I am putting some thing back and helping people who have been in the same situation as me. Soon I will be going on the wards twice a week at the Bradgate unit some time in May it will be a journey for me.

How my Bi-polar Disorder affects me now

26th March 2008, thankfully I am still married to Janet. She has seen me go through four nervous breakdowns, two of them in which we were married. We have been together ten years this year and married six of them. Janet is my rock and also my soul mate there's not many that come like her. I love her to bits and not many stand by you like she has done me. As they say through thick and thin. I would not be the man I am without her.

I have had thirteen years of mental health problems and I am now forty-six. My daughter comes to visit me every week and I play snooker once a week with a friend and every other week with my Cpn I enjoy it and it gets me out of the house. I am looking forward to the summer it makes me feel better, I have a big garden of which I grow vegetables in it; I also enjoy the big family barbeques that we have. I also enjoy walking I walk four times a week for an a hour it helps get the negative thoughts out of my system and I try to think more positive this time. I cannot believe that I have just shared thirteen years of my life experiences. We have come to the end of the book now. I hope you have enjoyed reading it as much as I have writing it.

I am happy with what I have got in life, I do struggle sometimes with the stigma but I suppose its because I want to play snooker at Willy Thorns snooker hall in the monthly handicaps.

Sometimes I feel like people give me a hard time or it just could be me. I seen some ex miners down town and they asked me what I was doing now. I have not worked for a long while but I cannot bring myself to tell them the truth. That I have been in an Asylum and that I have had five nervous breakdowns over the years. I wouldn't want to put them through it.

Sleep is the most important thing in life, I cannot sleep properly because of what has happened but also it could be my Bi-Polar Disorder. I roughly get five hours sleep in the winter, I am more active in the summer I also seem to get between six to seven hours sleep and try to keep myself busy as much as I can. Keep taking your medication I hope this is the last of my breakdowns but I know that I will still hit the hard times.

Never forget your past, but stop dwelling on it.

- There's never been a greatest thing in life than a touch of madness.

- Do not fall by the wayside.

- Fight Depression.

- Stay strong.

- Enjoy life.

www.ingramcontent.com/pod-product-compliance
Lightning Source LLC
Chambersburg PA
CBHW031213270326
41931CB00006B/555